O A P L
OXFORD AMERICAN PSYCHIATRY LIBRARY

Clinician's Guide to Psychiatric Care

D1617110

O A P L
OXFORD AMERICAN PSYCHIATRY LIBRARY

Clinician's Guide to Psychiatric Care

Edited by

Wei Jiang, MD

Associate Professor
Department of Psychiatry and Behavioral Sciences
Department of Internal Medicine
Duke University Medical Center, Durham, NC

Jane P. Gagliardi, MD

Assistant Clinical Professor
Department of Psychiatry and Behavioral Sciences
Department of Internal Medicine
Duke University Medical Center, Durham, NC

K. Ranga Krishnan, MD

Professor and Chairman
Department of Psychiatry and Behavioral Sciences
Duke University Medical Center, Durham, NC
Executive Vice Dean
NUS-GMS, Singapore

Executive Series Editor
Jeffrey A. Lieberman

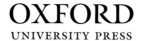

OXFORD
UNIVERSITY PRESS

OXFORD
UNIVERSITY PRESS

Oxford University Press, Inc., publishes works that further
Oxford University's objective of excellence
in research, scholarship, and education.

Oxford New York

Auckland Cape Town Dar es Salaam Hong Kong Karachi
Kuala Lumpur Madrid Melbourne Mexico City Nairobi
New Delhi Shanghai Taipei Toronto

With offices in

Argentina Austria Brazil Chile Czech Republic France Greece
Guatemala Hungary Italy Japan Poland Portugal Singapore
South Korea Switzerland Thailand Turkey Ukraine Vietnam

Published by Oxford University Press, Inc.
198 Madison Avenue, New York, New York 10016
www.oup.com

Oxford is a registered trademark of Oxford University Press

Library of Congress Cataloging-in-Publication Data

Clinician's guide to psychiatric care / edited by Wei Jiang,
Jane P. Gagliardi, K. Ranga Krishnan.
p. ; cm. — (Oxford American psychiatry library : OAPL)
Includes bibliographical references.
ISBN 978-0-19-536595-5

1. Psychiatry—Handbooks, manuals, etc. 2. Primary care (Medicine)—Handbooks,
manuals, etc. I. Jiang, Wei, 1953- II. Gagliardi, Jane P. III. Krishnan, K. Ranga Rama,
1956- IV. Series: Oxford American psychiatry library.
[DNLM: 1. Mental Disorders—therapy. 2. Psychiatry. WM 400 C6416 2008]
RC456.C58 2008
616.89—dc22   2008012488

9 8 7 6 5 4 3 2 1
Printed in the United States of America
on acid-free paper

Acknowledgment

We would like to acknowledge those who have contributed significantly to the establishment and success of the combined training program in Internal Medicine and Psychiatry at Duke University, namely Drs. G. Ralph Corey, Tana Grady, Greg Clary, Grace Thrall, and Diana McNeill, as well as past, present, and future trainees of this program. We also wish to acknowledge all of the authors who contributed their time and energy to this project.

Preface

Psychiatric illnesses are common among patients in nonpsychiatric settings. Approximately 50% of patients who visit primary care are significantly, or even primarily, affected by psychiatric problems. Many nonpsychiatric physicians or trainees encounter patients with psychiatric symptoms during their routine practice but may not feel comfortable managing psychiatric conditions. Psychiatric services, on the other hand, are not always readily available. Managing common psychiatric symptoms has therefore become an inevitable daily task for many primary care physicians (PCPs) and other nonpsychiatric practitioners.

The Duke Combined Medicine and Psychiatry clinicians are delighted to develop a manual book aiming to provide a concise, precise, and brisk overview on the recognition and management of major psychiatric problems such as depression, anxiety, suicidal statements, agitation, confusion, and other common presentations to providers in nonpsychiatric practice settings.

As a group of clinicians who care for patients hospitalized with significant medical and psychiatric comorbidities and who perform psychiatric consultation for medical and surgical patients, we believe the most active learning is accomplished when caring for patients. Therefore, most chapters in this book begin with a typical case presentation followed by an outline of commonly seen symptoms, bedside assessment, diagnosis and differentials, and treatment. This book especially focuses on differentials to help the nonpsychiatric practitioner gain a quick and easy grasp of common conditions, as well as suggestions for appropriate triage. Specific interventional considerations for unique psychiatric problems in patients with comorbid medical conditions are presented. In addition, several chapters address general psychiatric knowledge that is essential for every clinician, including the mental status examination and psychiatric diagnosis, psychopharmacology, overview of the practice of psychotherapy, principles of stress management, and neurocognitive and psychological assessment.

This book is not a comprehensive textbook, not a psychiatric practice guideline, and not a replacement for *DSM-IV* or *DSM-IV-TR*. This manual is designed chiefly to serve the nonpsychiatric clinician in the clinic or at the bedside of patients with psychiatric conditions. More comprehensive and sophisticated literature, including practice guidelines and some of the useful resources at the end of chapters, should be consulted for a more in-depth understanding of the various conditions discussed briefly in this book.

We hope this book serves as a friendly, handy, and reliable tool for nonpsychiatric clinicians, in particular primary care physicians and internists, in addressing common psychiatric issues that arise in the daily care of patients.

Contents

Contributors

Eric J. Christopher, MD

Assistant Professor, Department
of Psychiatry and Behavioral
Sciences
Clinical Associate
Department of Internal
Medicine
Duke University Medical Center
Durham, NC

Gregory Lunceford, MD

Assistant Director, Inpatient
Psychiatry Unit
Wellstar Psychiatry L.L.C.
Marietta, GA

Thomas R. Lynch, MD

Associate Professor
Department of Psychiatry and
Behavioral Sciences
Department of Psychology and
Neurosciences
Duke University Medical Center &
Duke University
Durham, NC

Guy G. Potter, PhD

Assistant Professor
Department of Psychiatry and
Behavioral Sciences
Division of Medical Psychology
Duke University
Durham, NC

Xavier Preud'homme, MD

Assistant Professor
Department of Psychiatry and
Behavioral Sciences
Department of Internal Medicine
Quantitative EEG and Sleep
Research Laboratory
Duke University Medical Center
Durham, NC

Pritham Raj, MD

Assistant Professor, Departments
of Internal Medicine and Psychiatry
Oregon Health & Science
University
Portland, OR
Clinical Associate, Department of
Psychiatry and Behavioral Science
Duke University Medical Center
Durham, NC

Yeshesvini Raman, MD

Clinical Associate
Department of Psychiatry and
Behavioral Sciences
Department of Internal Medicine
Duke University Medical Center
Durham, NC

Sarah Rivelli, MD

Clinical Associate
Department of Psychiatry and
Behavioral Sciences
Department of Internal Medicine
Duke University Medical Center
Durham, NC

Jon Seskevich, RN, BSN

Nurse Clinician
Advanced Clinical Practice
Department
Duke University Hospital
Duke University Medical Center
Durham, NC

Moria J. Smoski, PhD
Clinical Associate/Postdoctoral
Fellow
Department of Psychiatry and
Behavioral Sciences
Cognitive Behavioral Research and
Treatment Program
Duke University Medical Center
Durham, NC

Glen L. Xiong, MD
Assistant Clinical Professor
Department of Psychiatry and
Behavioral Sciences
Department of Internal Medicine
University of California, Davis
Sacramento, CA

Chapter 1

Communicating effectively with patients

Jane P. Gagliardi and Wei Jiang

Over a typical 40-year career, an average physician can expect to conduct about 200,000 patient interviews. In these interviews, patients and physicians exchange information about the patient that can be crucial not only for the physician–patient relationship but also for appropriate differential diagnosis formulation and treatment planning. In short, communication matters. Although many physicians feel communication skills to be intuitive, effective communication becomes more challenging in the face of pressures to shorten patient visits and cover more material in each encounter. Moreover, the art of communication is not consistently a priority in the formal education of clinicians, many of whom are uncomfortable handling patients' emotional concerns.

Good doctor–patient communication offers patients tangible benefits. Studies have shown significant positive associations between doctors' communication skills and patients' satisfaction,[1] as well as a positive correlation between effective communication and improved health outcomes (i.e., emotional health, resolution of symptoms, function, pain control, and physiological measures such as blood pressure and blood sugar concentration).[2] In other words, good communication improves patients' physical health.

What do patients want? The most common complaint from patients is that doctors do not listen to them. Patients want more and better information about their problem and the outcome, more openness about the side effects of treatment, relief of pain and emotional distress, and advice on what they can do for themselves.[3–5] (Refer also to Chapter 22, "Approaches to Stress Management.")

Empathic listening

Perhaps the most important skill to develop for effective communication is *empathic listening*. Empathic listening, also called active listening or reflective listening, is a way of listening and responding to another person that improves mutual understanding and trust. As patients become "health care consumers" and assume a more active role as participants in medical decision making, the traditional "parental" role of physicians is rendered obsolete. Patients want a doctor who communicates well and understands their needs, reflected in the fact that more lawsuits originate from patient dissatisfaction with physicians' interpersonal communication skills than from clinical competency.[6,7]

Empathic listening can provide several benefits, including the following:

- It builds trust and respect.
- It enables disputants to release their emotions.
- It reduces tension.
- It encourages the surfacing of information.
- It creates a safe environment that is conducive to collaborative problem-solving.

Being empathic

Empathy is the ability to project oneself into the personality of another person in order to better understand that person's emotions or feelings—putting oneself into the other person's shoes. Although it may appear trifling, any issue that a patient raises is a vital concern or problem to him or her. The goal of empathic listening is to convey the message of importance and validation through words and nonverbal behaviors, including body language, to encourage the speaker to fully express himself or herself. Empathic listening lets the speaker know the listener understands the problem and the feelings it evokes and is interested in being a resource to help solve the problem. The specific skills of being an empathic listener include the following:

- willingness to let the patient dominate the discussion;
- adopting a nonjudgmental, nondefensive stance;
- remaining attentive to what is being said;
- clarifying questions and restating what the listener perceives the speaker to be saying;
- being quiet and not interrupting (an immediate reply is not necessary; often patients in emotional distress are able to calm down if allowed to ventilate their feelings);
- asking open-ended questions; and
- being sensitive to the emotions being expressed by offering verbal or nonverbal support such as leaning forward, using facial expressions, using short verbal cues (e.g., "yes," "go on," "oh," "uh-huh," or "mmm"), and reflecting back on the substance and feelings being expressed.

Other effective communication skills

Acknowledging and validating the patient's concerns

Physicians may be tired of hearing complaints from certain patients, especially those with chronic pain demanding more pain medications, patients with multiple physical symptoms without identifiable pathological etiology, or those who are obsessed with their medical conditions. In many of these instances, the patients themselves are also frustrated, and a simple acknowledgment of this frustration can go a long way. A genuine statement such as "I can see how much you are suffering" or "It seems you are frustrated with what's going on" can reduce the tension and make the patient feel better. Even when the physician acknowledges, "I understand you feel poorly, though I am not sure we will be able to identify a clear cause," the patient will feel heard. In return, the physician will have a better chance of being able to discuss diagnostic limitations and issues with more honesty. The point of acknowledgment and validation is to let patients know that the physician understands they are individuals with particular experiences and perspectives who are affected by their symptoms.

Respecting the patient

Never discount a patient's experience, because it is real for the patient. Avoid saying things like "There is nothing wrong with you." Patients' perceptions play a significant role in the care physicians provide. Expressing open skepticism or doubts is unlikely to improve the patient–physician relationship. Even when working with a patient who is known to be malingering, simply "catching" the patient in his or her deceit is not the goal. Even in such an extreme case, "When a patient is found to be a malingerer, clinicians should tactfully and non-judgmentally present inconsistencies to the patient and offer a face-saving way out of the interaction."[8] Such an approach will minimize shame, hostility, and repulsion and will ultimately result in better health outcomes through the development of trust and rapport between the physician and the patient.

Appreciating the patient

American health care is evolving from physician-centered service to patient-centered service. Therefore, it is advisable to be grateful to the "health care customers" who are the patients. Small statements to patients and their families such as "I appreciate your coming to me with this," "I know it's hard to discuss these things," "I appreciate your making the effort to talk with me about this," and "Thanks for letting me know what is going on with you" will enhance rapport.

Following through

Although time constraints exist in busy practices, it is crucial to follow through with tasks. Patients who have lab tests or procedures appreciate knowing the results and participating in a discussion about implications and next steps. Patients referred for consultation or other services should be asked about their experiences, and the physician should respond appropriately (refer to Chapter 2, "When to Call for Psychiatric Help"). Making clear notes about what will be followed up on and discussed at the next visit is one way to be more effective and efficient. Returning patients' messages as promised also plays a significant role in effective communication.

The BATHE technique for emotionally challenging patients

The BATHE technique[9] is an open-ended questioning technique with an algorithm that has been suggested for use when the physician suspects there may be a psychological component to a patient's complaint. The BATHE technique divides the patient interview into the following components and was designed to fit smoothly into a 15-minute patient visit:

- **Background** ("Tell me what has been happening.")
- **Affect** ("How do you feel about that?")
- **Trouble** ("What's upsetting you most about it?")
- **Handling** ("How are you handling the situation?")
- **Empathy** ("That must have been difficult.")

Effective communication is a key element in adopting a patient-centered approach to providing appropriate medical care and to reducing adversarial clinician–patient relationships. By incorporating effective communication techniques into daily patient interactions, clinicians can decrease their malpractice risk. More importantly, clinicians with effective communication skills will be able to enjoy their patient interactions and work toward the goal of making a positive and effective impact on patient health outcomes without increasing the length of visits.

References

1. Ong LM, de Haes JC, Hoos AM, Lammes FB. Doctor-patient communication: a review of the literature. *Soc Sci Med.* 1995;40:903–918.

2. Stewart MA. Effective physician-patient communication and health outcomes: a review. *Can Med Assoc J.* 1995;152:1423–1433.

3. Sanchez-Menegay C, Stalder H. Do physicians take into account patients' expectations? *J Gen Intern Med.* 1994;9:404–406.

4. Laine C, Davidoff F, Lewis CE, et al. Important elements of outpatient care: a comparison of patients' and physicians' opinions. *Ann Intern Med.* 1996;125:640–645.

5. Roter DL, Steward M, Putnam SM, Lipkin M, Stiles W, Inui TS. Communication patterns of primary care physicians. *JAMA.* 1997;277:350–356.

6. Beckman HB, Markakis KM, Suchman AL, Frankel RM. The doctor-patient relationship and malpractice. *Arch Intern Med.* 1994;154:1365–1370.

7. Richards T. Chasms in communication. *BMJ.* 1990;301:1407–1408.

8. Adetunji BB, Mathews M, Williams A, Osinowo T, Oladinni O. Detection and management of malingering in a clinical setting. *Prim Psychiatry.* 2006;13:61–69.

9. Stuart MR, Lieberman JA. *The Fifteen-Minute Hour: Applied Psychotherapy for the Primary Care Physician.* Westport, CT: Praeger Publishers; 1993.

Chapter 2

When to call for psychiatric help

Wei Jiang and Jane P. Gagliardi

Clinical Scenario

Dr. J is seeing a middle-aged female patient in his clinic for the second time. The patient has a long history of Crohn's disease, with prominent complaints of abdominal pain and nausea. She has a history of multiple abdominal surgeries as well as a history of depression. She has been on methadone for chronic abdominal pain. Shortly into the clinic visit, she becomes tearful and tells Dr. J that she has been thinking about ending her life so she will not struggle with her Crohn's disease any more. Concerned, Dr. J brings up the possibility of sending the patient to see a psychiatrist. At this, the patient becomes upset, gets up, and pulls a pair of scissors out of her bag, stating she will stab anyone who tries to send her to see a "shrink."

Background

Questions of when to call for psychiatric help or when to refer a patient to a psychiatrist or psychiatric care may come to mind any time a patient reports psychiatric symptoms to the primary care provider or nonpsychiatric professional (PCP). It is well documented in the general medical setting that as many as 30% of patients have a diagnosable psychiatric disorder.[1–3] In the primary care and medical settings, there are numerous situations in which psychiatric manifestations go undetected. Among hospitalized patients, studies report great variability in the utilization of psychiatric consultation, ranging from a low of 1% to a high of 10%.[4,5] Delayed referral to psychiatric care may impair patients' recovery and overall outcomes. Prompt and appropriate referral to psychiatric care is a part of good medical practice. Nevertheless, there are no formal guidelines for referrals to psychiatric care.

Many factors may contribute to the ambiguous answer as to when and under what circumstances a patient needs psychiatric referral, including the PCP's beliefs or confidence level in caring for psychiatric illness; practice settings and availability of mental health referral; socioeconomic and environmental support available to patients; patients' ability to afford and access mental health care; and patients' beliefs and preferences regarding a highly stigmatized field of practice.[6] Combined with these factors, there is no clear evidence supporting definitive indications for psychiatric referral.[7–9] Given all of the above concerns, what follows is an experience-based recommendation for making appropriate referrals for psychiatric or mental health evaluation.

What requires mental health attention

Although most mental health problems come to the attention of PCPs and many are recognized and appropriately treated without ever coming to the attention of the mental health system, many conditions that PCPs encounter may warrant psychiatric referral. The common problems leading to requests for psychiatric consultation in the inpatient medical or surgical settings are summarized in the Academy of Psychosomatic Medicine's 1998 Practice Guidelines for Psychiatric Consultation in the General Medical Setting.[10]

Many conditions or illnesses that prompt psychiatric referral may not actually be psychiatric in origin. For instance, patients adjusting to AIDS or HIV infection, terminal illness, dying, or bereavement; patients who need determination of capacity or attention to other forensic or ethical issues; or patients who have difficulties with pain management may all be appropriate for psychiatric referral. In many instances, the reason for initiating consultation may be quite different from the formal psychiatric diagnosis resulting from a thorough psychiatric evaluation, and more serious problems are frequently identified by the consultant. Hence, a good rule of the thumb is to ask for psychiatric assistance whenever the symptoms presented are puzzling or cause concern, or any time the PCP thinks psychiatric assistance may be useful.

Where to find psychiatric help

Psychiatric care is no longer accomplished only by solo psychiatrists and is not always easy to find in one umbrella agency. There are a number of possible providers of mental health evaluation and care, including general psychiatrists, subspecialty psychiatrists, psychologists, and licensed clinical social workers with mental health experience, and a variety of community organizations and agencies with ties to the mental health setting. The most important step for PCPs to appropriately refer patients for psychiatric services is to know the available local resources, including emergency evaluation services (frequently available in emergency departments or local mental health entities run through the county or state), inpatient psychiatric facilities, social services, and the availability of counseling and therapy in the area. Ideally, a PCP would interact with a consistent liaison psychiatrist on a regular basis to establish rapport and a strong referral pattern, but this luxury is rare for many reasons, including differences in mental health coverage across insurance carriers and the fact that many patients impaired by mental health issues are uninsured. In an emergent situation such as that presented in the vignette involving a patient who is in danger of harming herself or who threatens other people's safety, it is important to contact local police to determine local laws governing the involuntary petitioning of patients for immediate psychiatric evaluation, and to become familiar with whom to call in an emergent situation.

Making an appropriate psychiatric referral

To optimize psychiatric evaluation and treatment, referral should be timely and as explicit as possible. For instance, the patient presented in the clinical scenario provides an indication for immediate (emergent) psychiatric referral and would clearly benefit from long-term outpatient psychiatric care. First of all, assuming her first visit to Dr. J had proceeded smoothly, the patient's dysphoria and agitated mood as well as her suicidal comment and threatening behavior during the second visit are concerning for acute distress. The differential for her distress is broad and includes the stress of a new environment, substance intoxication or withdrawal, family conflicts, stress resulting from exacerbation of her underlying medical condition, relapsing depressive disorder, or any combination of such factors. **The presence of suicidal or homicidal ideation with intent and means to hurt oneself or another person is an emergent situation requiring mental health evaluation on an emergency basis, including involuntary petition if the patient is unwilling to cooperate.**

The patient's presentation also illustrates several potential issues that may be best addressed in long-term outpatient psychiatric care with a regular provider. Although it is likely on emergency referral that she will be referred for inpatient psychiatric hospitalization, most inpatient psychiatric services currently operate on a model emphasizing acute stabilization and crisis management, with brief hospitalizations being the norm and appropriate outpatient follow-up a must. Patients with chronic psychiatric conditions are best served by regular follow-up in the outpatient setting. The patient presented in the vignette takes methadone for chronic pain and still has complaints of abdominal pain and nausea. Methadone is not routinely used for pain control, so its use raises a red flag for opiate dependence and abuse. Approximately 90% of patients with opiate dependence have additional major psychiatric comorbidities, such as major depressive disorder, alcohol use disorders, antisocial personality disorder, and anxiety disorders. These patients usually have limited coping skills and tend to react negatively to increased life stress. Her chronic abdominal symptoms may be at least partially somatic. With her mental health issues taken care of by a psychiatrist, particularly with good communication between the PCP and the psychiatrist, the patient will be better served, and ideally there will be less stress on the relationship between the patient and the PCP. In this particular case, referral to a pain management clinic incorporating psychiatric and/or psychological services might be a good option if such exists in the local area.

To best assist PCPs in making proper psychiatric referrals, Table 2.1 outlines conditions requiring a referral and the particular psychiatric service best suited to the conditions.

Many patients may interpret a psychiatric referral as abandonment by the PCP; this can hurt the patient–physician relationship and reduce the patient's ability to cooperate with treatment plans. Because of the

Table 2.1 Indications for specific psychiatric referral

Conditions	Where to refer
Patient who presents with *active* suicidal ideation or increased intensity of chronic suicidal ideation and/or has plan of harming self	Emergent or inpatient psychiatry May require legal proceedings—the patient's presentation to the ER or crisis center should be ensured by legal proceedings
Patient who presents with *acute or active* homicidal ideation	Emergent or inpatient psychiatry May require legal proceedings—the patient's presentation to the ER or crisis center should be ensured by legal proceedings
Patient who presents with *acute* delusions, hallucinations, agitation, or confusion	ER or inpatient psychiatry
Patient who requests assisted suicide or euthanasia	Emergent psychiatry to evaluate for depression. In this case, the psychiatrist may serve as a liaison between the patient and the health care team, serving to clarify goals and preferences for both. The consultant will need information about the patient's diagnosis, expected prognosis, risks and benefits of ongoing treatment plan, and any other issues that have arisen during the illness.
Patient who refuses proper care from PCP for a life-threatening medical or surgical condition	Emergency psychiatric evaluation for decision-making capacity. The consultant will need information about the patient's diagnosis, expected prognosis, risks and benefits of proposed treatments or interventions, and risks and benefits of proceeding without the proposed treatments or interventions.
Patient who presents with chronic and/or passive suicidal ideation (decreased will to live)	Prompt referral to outpatient psychiatry
Patient who presents with chronic and/or passive homicidal ideation	Prompt referral to outpatient psychiatry
Patient who presents with psychiatric symptoms and has history of violent behaviors	Prompt referral to outpatient psychiatry
Patient who presents with *chronic* psychotic symptoms, agitation, or confusions but no acutely life-threatening behaviors	Outpatient psychiatry
PCP is uncertain about the psychiatric diagnosis	Outpatient psychiatry
Patient whom the PCP is not comfortable managing psychiatrically Certain pharmacologic therapies, including lithium, monoamine oxidase inhibitors, or psychotropic medications in the setting of multiple other medications, may be best managed with a psychiatrist following the patient regularly.	Outpatient psychiatry

Table 2.1 *continued*

Conditions	Where to refer
Patients with a history of major psychiatric disorders, such as schizophrenia, bipolar disorder or mania, obsessive-compulsive disorder and other severe anxiety disorders, multiple previous suicide attempts, polysubstance abuse that is ongoing, inability to function socially, etc.	Outpatient psychiatry
Patient who is unresponsive to therapy with first-line antidepressants	Outpatient psychiatry
Patient who develops significant side effects from psychotropics	Outpatient psychiatry
Patient who takes multiple psychotropics	Outpatient psychiatry
Patient who presents with physical symptoms not well explained by medical etiology	Outpatient psychiatry
Patient who presents with very low weight and is not concerned	Outpatient psychiatry
Patient who is not compliant with recommended interventions	Outpatient psychiatry
Patient who presents with substance abuse or dependence	Substance abuse treatment programs
Patient who presents with evidence of being abused	Adult Protective Services
Physician suspects abuse or unsafe treatment of a child	Immediate referral to Child Protective Services
Patient whose family is dysfunctional	Social service and/or psychological counseling
Patient who is unable to function socially	Social service and/or psychological counseling

high prevalence of stigma against psychiatric practice and lack of psychological insight, it will be very helpful for PCPs to follow these suggestions:

1. Confidently and enthusiastically inform the patient about the referral (and rationale) for psychiatric evaluation or intervention. Ask about and listen to the patient's opinion or concerns about the referral.
2. Contact the psychiatric service and discuss specific concerns or reason for the request.
3. Provide the psychiatric service with any information about previous providers, demographic information, or any ongoing medical issues about the patient. Provide as much psychosocial information as possible to the consultant.
4. If it is not an emergent referral, establish an actual appointment for the patient. Mental health practices can be difficult for first-time patients to successfully navigate, particularly given the stigma of mental health and potential impairment due to the patient's mental health issues. Follow up to see whether the patient kept the appointment.

5. Follow up on and review with the patient his or her experience with the psychiatric referral.
6. Work with the psychiatric provider to coordinate care, particularly when medications are involved. Many psychiatric medications have the potential to interact with medications routinely prescribed in primary care practices.

References

1. Strain JJ. Needs for psychiatry in the general hospital. *Hosp Commun Psychiatry.* 1982;33:996–1001.

2. vonAmmon Cavanaugh S, Wettstein RM. Emotional and cognitive dysfunction associated with medical disorders. *J Psychosom Res.* 1989;33:505–514.

3. Spitzer RL, Kroenke K, Linzer M, et al. Health-related quality of life in primary care patients with mental disorders. Results from the PRIME-MD 1000 Study. *JAMA.* 1995;274:1511–1517.

4. Pablo RY, Lamarre CJ. Psychiatric consultations on a general hospital. *Can J Psychiatry.* 1988;33:224–230.

5. Wallen J, Pincus HA, Goldman HH, Marcus SE. Psychiatric consultations in short-term general hospitals. *Arch Gen Psychiatry.* 1987;44:163–168.

6. U.S. Surgeon General. *Mental Health: A Report of the Surgeon General.* Rockville, MD: U.S. Public Health Service, U.S. Department of Health and Human Services; 1999.

7. Verhaak PF, Tijhuis MA. Psychosocial problems in primary care: some results from the Dutch National Study of Morbidity and Interventions in General Practice. *Soc Sci Med.* 1992;35:105–110.

8. Adeyemi JD, Olonade PO, Amira CO. Attitude to psychiatric referral: a study of primary care physicians. *Nigerian Postgrad Med J.* 2002;9:53–58.

9. Trude S, Stoddard JJ. Referral gridlock: primary care physicians and mental health services. *J Gen Intern Med.* 2003;18:442–449.

10. Bronheim HE, Fulop G, Kunkel EJ, et al. The Academy of Psychosomatic Medicine practice guidelines for psychiatric consultation in the general medical setting. The Academy of Psychosomatic Medicine. *Psychosomatics.* 1998;39:S8–30.

Chapter 3

Mental status examination and diagnosis

Eric J. Christopher

The Mental Status Examination (MSE) is the fundamental diagnostic tool of psychiatry. It is used to objectively examine and describe the present mental status and function of a patient. The MSE also provides a way to assess a patient longitudinally and is an essential element of assessments done by mental health care providers, including psychiatrists, psychologists, and social workers. As there are no laboratory tests to confirm the presence of psychiatric disorders, a thorough MSE enables clinicians to develop a differential diagnosis. All health care providers should be aware of the elements of the MSE so they do not neglect major psychiatric conditions and are able to effectively communicate with mental health providers.

The Mental Status Examination

To make a diagnosis and facilitate communication with other mental health professionals, it is important to understand the individual components and descriptors of the MSE. Key elements of the MSE include the following:

1. appearance and general behavior;
2. level of consciousness;
3. attitude, speech;
4. psychomotor activity;
5. mood and affect;
6. thought process and content;
7. perceptions;
8. suicide and homicide assessment;
9. insight and judgment;
10. cognition; and
11. abstract reasoning.

Table 3.1 gives more detailed descriptors and possible disorders involved in each of the MSE elements.

The MSE describes the current, observed mental state of the patient. Because there are many sensitive pieces of information involved in a thorough psychiatric interview and MSE, it is preferable to perform the examination in the absence of any family members or friends, since patients

Table 3.1 Outline of mental status examination

MSE item	Possible descriptors	Possible disorders
Appearance	Disheveled, casual, well-dressed, appearing older or younger than stated age, malodorous, restless, lacking eye contact, etc.	Unkempt appearance in psychotic disorders; excessive jewelry or makeup in mania or histrionic personality; tired, listless appearance in depression
General behavior	Cooperative, hostile, aggressive, etc.	Agitation in substance intoxication; suspiciousness in psychotic disorders
Level of consciousness	Alert, stuporous, comatose	Catatonia may be present in psychotic disorders; fluctuating level of consciousness in delirium
Speech	Volume, tone, rate, latency, lack of speech or muteness	Loud, rapid speech in mania; increased latency may signify psychotic disorder
Psychomotor	Normal, tremors, hyper- or hypoactive, paresis, weak, other abnormal movement	Catatonia may be present in psychotic disorders; hyperactivity in substance intoxication, mania; decreased movements (psychomotor retardation) in depressive disorders
Mood	**Examinee's perception** of current emotional state: happy, sad, mad, angry, upset, excited, depressed, anxious (e.g., patient's response to question: "How's your mood?")	
Affect	**Examiner's interpretation** of patient's current mood state, with notation as to whether it seems appropriate or inappropriate to a patient's stated mood. For example, a patient who says she is sad and is crying during the interview shows **mood congruence**, whereas a patient who laughs at an inappropriate time demonstrates **mood-incongruent** affect.	Elevated, expansive affect in mania; flat or constricted affect in depressive disorders
Thought process	Form and process of thought; conveys the patient's ability to "stay on track." Normal is logical and goal-directed. Abnormal descriptors include tangential (unable to stay on track), circumferential (eventually gets to the point around a circuitous route), disorganized, confused, flight of ideas, loosening of associations, thought-blocking.	Disorganized in psychotic disorders; tangential in some cognitive disorders; circumferential in some anxiety or obsessive-compulsive disorders; flight of ideas in mania

Table 3.1 *continued*

MSE item	Possible descriptors	Possible disorders
Thought content	Abnormal perceptions, including illusions or hallucinations (auditory [noises or voices], visual, or tactile), delusions (fixed, false beliefs that are not explained by cultural viewpoint), thought insertion or thought withdrawal	Mainly seen in psychotic disorders
Suicidality/ homicidality	Patient's attitude regarding harm to self or others. **It is not safe to assume lack of either suicidality or homicidality in any patient—this must be specifically asked about.** "Have you had any thoughts about ending your life or harming anyone else?" is one way to screen. Another is to ask how the patient feels about being alive or whether he or she has considered that he or she would be better off dead. Asking about suicide and homicide does *not* make a patient "prone" to either action.	
Insight and judgment	Is the patient aware of his or her condition (insight)? How appropriate are his or her actions (judgment)?	
Cognition	Orientation, memory, etc. (see Table 13.3 for details)	See Table 13.3 for details

will not always feel comfortable disclosing thought content or suicidality/homicidality in the presence of family or friends.

Several other factors must be attended to during the psychiatric interview. Patients should be made to feel at ease and supported. This will help in gaining the most information from the patient. Questions should be open-ended to allow the patient to express his or her feelings. It is important to obtain information in a nonjudgmental manner, especially when asking about physical and sexual abuse, as well as substance use.

The potential for violence exists in any clinical interaction, whether or not a psychiatric disorder is present. Patients can react violently for a number of reasons, including fear, active delirium, or substance intoxication. In addition, some patients can be intimidating or hostile. The clinician should assess continuously for the presence of any behaviors that may indicate increasing patient distress or agitation (e.g., roving gaze as if trying to escape; a blank, intimidating stare; increasing respiratory rate; and posturing in an aggressive manner). Some patients will "shut down" and have psychomotor retardation before becoming violent.

Clinicians can protect themselves with a few preventive measures. The examiner should sit between the patient and the door so he or she has an escape route if needed. If a patient is known to be violent or is behaviorally disinhibited, hospital police or security should be present *before* the interview so they will be available for immediate assistance if needed.

Bedside cognitive screening

For a thorough MSE, at least one cognitive screen should be performed. This provides "hard data" as well as a basis for comparison. Many bedside examinations can be used to either quantify the severity of impairment or help in the longitudinal assessment of the patient, particularly in cases of delirium and dementia. The best-known examination of this type is the Folstein Mini-Mental State Examination (MMSE).[1] It is simple to perform and usually readily accepted by patients. Although it may appear simple, it is important to put the patient at ease and adopt a nonjudgmental stance. For example, telling a patient, "Now I am going to ask you some questions. Some of them are easy and some are hard; just try your best" can alleviate some of the anxiety that patients may experience when being assessed in this way. External interruptions should be minimized. Ideally, the patient should be examined alone, without family or friends present—family members sometimes try to provide correct answers, patients may feel embarrassed or frustrated if family members see them doing poorly on a simple cognitive test, and family members may be shocked to find out how impaired their loved one is.

The MMSE provides a broad picture of cognitive function. It has varying sensitivity and specificity across various educational, racial, and socio-economic backgrounds. In general, any score less than 25 out of 30 in a high school graduate is concerning. The MMSE is not a screen for mild impairment in cognition, which requires more detailed, formal memory testing, usually conducted by a neuropsychologist (refer to Chapter 23, "Neurocognitive and Psychological Assessment").

Other screening examinations are used with objective scales to help determine cognitive domains such as memory and include the word lists, Wechsler Memory Scale, Logical Memory, and Benton Visual Retention Test. (Other cognitive screening tests include Clock Drawing and the Montreal Cognitive Assessment [MoCA].[2]) Additional screening tests that provide "hard data" on the presence and severity of individual psychiatric disorders exist. Self-rated or examiner-observed rating scales include the Hamilton Depression Scale (HDRS), Beck Depression Inventory (BDI), Young Mania Rating Scale (YMRS), Hamilton Rating Scale for Anxiety (HAM-A), Yale-Brown Obsessive Compulsive Scale (Y-BOCS), Positive and Negative Symptom Scale for Schizophrenia (PANSS), Abnormal Involuntary Movement Scale (AIMS), and many others.

Diagnosis

Once history, background, MSE, and collateral information have been obtained, a psychiatric diagnosis can be made. The following chapters will discuss different conditions and their diagnosis. Psychiatric assessments are made on a "multi-axial" hierarchy to encompass the biopsychosocial situation of the patient, since psychiatric conditions involve the total person. In forming this assessment, five domains are considered in the final diagnosis (Axis I through Axis V).[3] Axis I represents "clinical syndromes" or other psychiatric "conditions that are a focus of attention or treatment"[4]—in other words, the "diagnosis" that brings the patient to psychiatric (or other mental health) attention. Developmental delays (such as mental retardation) and personality disorders are excluded from Axis I. Axis II, which includes personality disorders and mental retardation, typically takes a bit more effort to discern. Most of the time, making a confident Axis II diagnosis requires more than one or two visits. Axis III indicates medical problems that may contribute to or be influenced by the mental health disorder or treatment of the individual who has developed the Axis I diagnosis. Axis III includes a wide variety of medical problems.[5] Axis IV consists of "psychosocial and environmental problems that may affect the diagnosis, treatment, and prognosis of mental disorders." Axis V is designated to provide a "Global Assessment of Functioning," to quantify the effectiveness of adaptation at given relevant points in time.[5]

References

1. Folstein MF, Folstein SE, McHugh PR. "Mini-mental state." A practical method for grading the cognitive state of patients for the clinician. *J Psychiatr Res.* 1975;12(3):189–198.

2. Nasreddine ZS, Phillips NA, Bédirian V, et al. The Montreal Cognitive Assessment, MoCA: a brief screening tool for mild cognitive impairment. *J Am Geriatr Soc.* 2005;53(4):695–699.

3. American Psychiatric Association. *Diagnostic and Statistical Manual of Mental Disorders, 4th ed., Text Revision.* Washington, DC: American Psychiatric Association; 2000.

4. American Psychiatric Association. *Diagnostic and Statistical Manual of Mental Disorders, 3rd ed.* Washington, DC: American Psychiatric Association; 1980.

5. Oken D. Multiaxial diagnosis and the psychosomatic model of disease. *Psychosom Med.* 2000;62:171–175.

Chapter 4

An overview of psychopharmacologic therapies

Jane P. Gagliardi

Psychiatric diagnosis and treatment have been revolutionized by the development of psychotropic medications. When used appropriately in patients who meet the criteria for specific psychiatric disturbances, medications can be very helpful. It is important that the patient undergo a sufficiently complete psychiatric interview to accurately diagnose the targeted disorder (refer to Chapter 3, "Mental Status Examination and Diagnosis"). When considering starting medications for a psychiatric disorder, it is important to have an honest and up-front discussion with the patient, including rationale, expected benefits, and anticipated side effects. Such a discussion can be crucial to patient adherence and satisfaction. Patients should be followed closely when new medications are being started, and nonpsychiatric providers should have a low threshold for requesting psychiatric consultation for diagnostic clarification or medication consultation. In such cases, consultation may consist of one or two visits, with the primary care provider continuing to provide continuity care and medication management once the treatment has been clarified.

General principles of psychopharmacology

There are a few principles that apply to the prescription of most psychoactive medications.

Accurate diagnosis

Diagnosis is an important factor in choosing the correct psychopharmacologic treatment. A patient with symptoms of depression (refer to Chapter 7, "The Patient with Depressive Symptoms") may have straightforward major depressive disorder, in which case treatment with a selective serotonin reuptake inhibitor (SSRI) may be effective. However, SSRI therapy can be counterproductive in patients who have underlying bipolar disorder, and it is important to screen for symptoms of mania before initiating the medication (refer to Chapter 8, "The Patient with Manic Symptoms").

Informed consent

Informed consent is an important process in the prescription of any medication but is particularly important when considering medication therapy for psychiatric indications. Studies show that patient adherence to psychotropic medications is low, and factors such as stigma, cost, and side effects may all play a role.[1] It is a good idea to determine the patient's attitude toward taking medications and to discuss possible barriers before initiating treatment with a psychoactive medication. Discuss the indication for the medication, anticipated effectiveness, typical time course to symptom improvement, and specific side effects with patients before initiating medications. An open attitude and honest discussion about the risks, benefits, and rationale of suggested treatment may enhance the physician–patient relationship and facilitate adherence to the treatment plan.

Pharmacodynamic interactions

Most psychoactive medications are metabolized by the liver through the cytochrome P450 (CYP450) enzyme system. Many medications, food, herbal remedies, and substances may be substrates, inducers, or inhibitors of specific CYP450 isoenzymes, and clinically significant pharmacodynamic interactions through the CYP450 enzyme system may result. This may be a particular issue in patients who take other medications or patients who take herbal remedies without informing their physician. It is therefore critical to maintain awareness of patients' use of medications and other remedies. In many cases it is possible to select a medication based on the least possible pharmacodynamic interactions. The Web site http://medicine.iupui .edu/flockhart/clinlist.htm provides information about CYP isoenzymes and medications metabolized through them.[2]

Psychopharmacological agents cross the placental barrier

Because psychiatric illness affects reproductive-aged women, and because most of the teratogenic effect of a psychoactive substance will manifest in the first trimester—a time when many women are not aware they are pregnant—it is important to remember that psychoactive medications cross the placental barrier and may cause problems in fetal development or the perinatal period.[3] For this reason, all women with intact reproductive systems should be counseled extensively regarding teratogenicity and effective birth control options *before* starting psychiatric medications. Optimally, the physician or provider will counsel and collaborate with female patients to choose the safest medications at the lowest effective doses *before* the patient seeks to become pregnant.

Familiarity with use

This is an important factor in the safe and effective prescription of psychotropic medications for reasons of informed consent and pharmacodynamic interactions as well as for reasons of safety and predictability of patient response. Therefore, the nonpsychiatric provider should initially become familiar with a few psychiatric medications and use these as first-line agents, then expand his or her knowledge about other psychotropic medications.

SSRIs are commonly prescribed for depressive and anxiety disorders, and many patients in nonpsychiatric practices will present with these disorders, so it makes sense to become comfortable prescribing various SSRIs and monitoring for effectiveness and side effects (refer to Chapter 7, "The Patient with Depressive Symptoms," and Chapter 9, "The Patient with Symptoms of Anxiety").

Psychiatric referral is sometimes the safest option. Though it makes sense for nonpsychiatric providers to become familiar with at least a few SSRIs and to be comfortable with their use and monitoring parameters, medications such as tricyclic antidepressants (TCAs) and monoamine oxidase inhibitors (MAOIs) have narrow therapeutic windows and may be best managed by psychiatric specialists. It is still important for nonpsychiatric providers to have some familiarity with possible interactions/adverse effects so that patients may be appropriately monitored.

Medications do not always play the most important role in the treatment of psychiatric disorders

The best treatment for a particular psychiatric disorder may involve pharmacotherapy, psychotherapy, or a combination (refer to Chapter 21, "Overview of the Practice of Psychotherapy"). Patients who fail to respond to usual measures should be referred to a psychiatric provider for further evaluation and management, including clarification of the diagnosis and optimization of therapy.

Treatment of depression

Medications and doses that are commonly used in the treatment of depression are summarized in Table 4.1.[1]

Table 4.1 Medications used to treat depression and anxiety disorders

Drug name[1]	Usual starting dose[2]	Usual effective daily dose
Selective serotonin reuptake inhibitors (antidepressant and antianxiety)[3]		
Citalopram	10 to 20 mg once daily	20 to 60 mg
Escitalopram	10 mg once daily	10 to 20 mg
Fluoxetine	10 to 20 mg once daily	20 to 80 mg
Fluvoxamine[4]	50 mg once daily	200 to 300 mg (divided bid or tid)
Paroxetine	10 to 20 mg once daily	10 to 50 mg
Controlled release	12.5 to 25 mg once daily	25 to 62.5 mg
Sertraline	12.5 to 50 mg once daily	25 to 200 mg
Serotonin-norepinephrine reuptake inhibitors[3] (antidepressant and antianxiety)		
Duloxetine	40 to 60 mg once daily	60 to 120 mg (no data to support 120 mg)

Table 4.1 *continued*

Drug name[1]	Usual starting dose[2]	Usual effective daily dose
Venlafaxine	25 mg tid	75 to 225 mg (divided bid or tid)
Extended release	37.5 to 75 mg once daily	75 to 225 mg
Bupropion[5]	100 mg bid	300 to 450 mg (not to exceed 150 mg/dose)
Sustained release	150 mg once daily	300 to 400 mg (divided bid)
Extended release	150 mg once daily	150 to 450 mg (300 mg usually effective)
Mirtazapine	15 mg once at bedtime	15 to 45 mg
Trazodone	50 mg tid	150 to 400 mg (divided bid or tid)
Tricyclic antidepressants[6] (antidepressant and antianxiety)		
Amitriptyline	25 to 75 mg at bedtime	75 to 200 mg (hs or divided bid)
Amoxapine	50 mg twice daily	200 to 300 mg (hs or divided bid)
Desipramine	50 to 75 mg once or divided	100 to 200 mg (hs or divided bid)
Doxepin	50 to 75 mg once or divided	75 to 150 mg (hs or divided bid/tid)
Imipramine	50 to 100 mg once or divided	100 to 200 mg (hs or divided bid to qid)
Maprotiline	25 mg tid	75 to 150 mg (hs or divided tid)
Nortriptyline	25 to 50 mg once or divided	50 to 150 mg (hs or divided bid)
Protriptyline	5 to 10 mg tid	20 to 60 mg (divided tid)
Trimipramine	25 mg tid	100 to 150 mg (divided tid)
MAO inhibitors[7] (antidepressant and antianxiety)		
Isocarboxazid	10 mg bid	20 to 40 mg (divided bid)
Phenelzine	15 mg tid	60 to 90 mg (divided tid)
Selegiline (transdermal)	6 mg/24 hours topically	6 to 12 mg/24 hours[8]
Tranylcypromine	30 mg divided bid or tid	30 to 60 mg (divided bid or tid)
Benzodiazepines[9,10] (used for treatment of anxiety)		
Alprazolam[11]	0.25 to 0.5 mg tid	1 to 4 mg (divided tid or qid)
Chlordiazepoxide	5 to 25 mg tid	50 to 100 mg (divided tid or qid)
Clorazepate	7.5 to 15 mg at bedtime	15 to 60 mg (divided bid or tid)
Diazepam[12]	5 mg bid or tid	5 to 30 mg (divided bid or tid)
Lorazepam[13]	1 to 2 mg divided bid or tid	2 to 6 mg (divided bid or tid)
Oxazepam[14]	10 mg tid	30 to 60 mg (divided tid or qid)
Other medications (used for treatment of anxiety)		
Buspirone	7.5 mg bid	15 to 30 mg (divided bid or tid)
Hydroxyzine[15]	12.5 to 50 mg up to qid	50 to 200 mg (divided bid or qid)
Meprobamate[16]	200 to 300 mg tid or qid	1200 to 2400 mg (divided tid or qid)

It is important to screen patients for lifetime history of mania before initiating an antidepressant of any class, and patients started on medication for depression should be monitored frequently (e.g., weekly) at the beginning of treatment to assess for agitation or the development of suicidality.

[1] Though not approved, many patients may take over-the-counter remedies such as St. John's wort, which does have evidence for effectiveness in mild to moderate depression. It is important to screen for such use, as serotonergic potentiation may result in a tendency toward serotonin syndrome.

[2] Use the lower starting dose in elderly patients or patients with anxiety disorders.

[3] SSRIs have been associated with increased risk of bleeding due to their inhibition of platelet function. Paroxetine and fluoxetine have the most CYP450 isoenzyme–mediated interactions and should be used cautiously in combination with other medications. SSRIs and SNRIs have been associated with an increased risk of hyponatremia, particularly in elderly patients. Epidemiologic studies have highlighted a possible risk for osteoporotic fracture with SSRIs, though there are no good prospective data and there is convincing evidence that untreated depression itself may cause osteoporosis.

[4] Not approved for use in depression.

[5] Bupropion is not effective in anxiety disorders.

[6] Most serum tricyclic concentrations can be monitored; narrow therapeutic window for safety. Lowest effective dose should be used. Obtain baseline ECG. Avoid in post-I patients or patients with AV conduction block. Psychiatric consultation may be helpful.

[7] Narrow therapeutic index; oral formulations require tyramine-restricted diet; need to make sure patient has been off other serotonergic agents for at least 2 weeks (longer for longer-half-life medications such as fluoxetine). Titration should be slow, keeping in mind patient tolerance of the medication, side effects, and potential adverse effects. Lowest effective dose should be used. Psychiatric consultation may be helpful.

[8] Higher doses of transdermal selegiline require tyramine-restricted diet.

[9] Benzodiazepines not considered best long-term medication for anxiety disorder. Potential for cognitive slowing, abuse, and addiction limits their use. Potential for life-threatening withdrawal syndrome and seizures with abrupt discontinuation.

[10] Long-acting benzodiazepines are federally prohibited for use in residents of long-term care facilities unless short-acting agents have failed.

[11] Rapid onset and offset; high abuse/addiction potential.

[12] Federal guidelines set 5 mg daily maximum in long-term care facility residents.

[13] Federal guidelines set 2 mg daily maximum in long-term care facility residents.

[14] Federal guidelines set 30 mg daily maximum in long-term care facility residents.

[15] Long-term use not recommended; federal guidelines set 50 mg daily maximum in long-term care facility residents. Anticholinergic effects may be detrimental to cognition.

[16] Federal guidelines set 600 mg daily maximum in long-term care facility residents.

The response rate for each individual agent is 40% to 60%. The time course for effective response to a dose of antidepressant medication is usually 2 to 6 weeks.[4] Antipsychotic medication should be added in cases of severe depression with features of psychosis, which may also prompt referral to a psychiatrist for further evaluation and management.[5]

When starting medications for depression, it is important to ascertain the severity of illness. It is also important to screen patients for lifetime history of mania (refer to Chapter 3, "Mental Status Examination and Diagnosis," and Chapter 8, "The Patient with Manic Symptoms"). All antidepressant medications have the potential to induce mania in patients with previously undisclosed or undiagnosed bipolar disorder, and patients should be closely monitored following initiation of antidepressant medications.

The patient should follow up with the prescribing physician at close intervals (about a week after initiating and then at least monthly thereafter)[6] to monitor for the development of any worsening anxiety or restlessness, suicidal ideation, psychotic features, or other new concerns and to rule out the presence of suicidal thoughts or plans. Psychiatric consultation is indicated in cases of new or active suicidal ideation (refer to Chapter 2, "When to Call for Psychiatric Help"). Referral is also recommended for patients requesting electroconvulsive therapy or other somatic therapies for depression, including vagus nerve stimulation or transcranial magnetic resonance stimulation, and patients with severe depression, psychotic features, bipolar depression, pregnancy, or other complicating factors.

SSRIs (fluoxetine, paroxetine, sertraline, citalopram, and escitalopram) are usually first-line agents in the treatment of depression. The serotonin-norepinephrine reuptake inhibitors (SNRIs) venlafaxine and duloxetine and other antidepressants (bupropion and mirtazapine) are also useful in the treatment of major depressive disorder. Older agents (TCAs and MAOIs), as well as the newer transdermal delivery of the selective MAOI selegiline, are also useful in cases of depression, particularly when it is refractory or severe. These older medications and augmentation strategies such as lithium, a second class of antidepressant, antipsychotics, or thyroid hormone are sometimes employed, especially in cases of treatment-resistant depression, though patients requiring such treatments will benefit from the ongoing input of a psychiatrist. There are few prospective studies of augmentation strategies.[7]

Treatment of anxiety disorders

Medications and doses that are commonly used in the treatment of anxiety are also summarized in Table 4.1.[1]

Although benzodiazepines are frequently prescribed for patients with anxiety symptoms, the best long-term pharmacological management for patients with anxiety disorder is an antidepressant,[8] in which case it is still important to screen patients for lifetime history of mania. The full effect of SSRIs in anxiety disorder may take several weeks. In cases of refractory panic disorder, TCAs or MAOIs are sometimes effective. When starting antidepressant therapy for an anxiety disorder, a good rule of thumb is to start at the lowest possible dose to minimize the initial jitteriness that may accompany antidepressant initiation—patients with anxiety disorders are particularly prone to this side effect and should be counseled to expect it.

Psychotherapy should be considered at least as part of a combination treatment for social anxiety, post-traumatic stress disorder, panic disorder, and generalized anxiety disorder when patients are able to access therapy. Some anxiety disorders, such as specific phobias, are not particularly responsive to medications—in these cases, psychotherapy is a mainstay of effective treatment (refer to Chapter 21, "Overview of the Practice of Psychotherapy"). In cases of severe anxiety disorder such as obsessive-compulsive disorder or post-traumatic stress disorder, higher target doses of antidepressants are sometimes required.

Benzodiazepines are effective anxiolytics but are optimally used in the short term or during SSRI up-titration, particularly given their potential for cognitive impairment and addiction. Several anticonvulsants, including gabapentin and tiagabine, have been used off-label with limited evidence as alternatives to benzodiazepines. Buspirone is sometimes prescribed for patients with generalized anxiety disorder and can be helpful, though frequently patients who have been treated with antidepressants and benzodiazepines will report little to no effect from buspirone. Patients with performance anxiety are frequently responsive to low doses of nonselective beta blockers such as propranolol before performances.

Treatment of bipolar disorder

A number of medications are approved for the treatment of bipolar disorder; they are summarized in Table 4.2.[1] Lithium is a good first-line treatment for bipolar disorder, but anticonvulsants such as valproic acid and carbamazepine are also effective. A number of second-generation (atypical) antipsychotic drugs are used in the acute and maintenance treatment of bipolar disorder, particularly mania or mixed episodes. Anticonvulsants with lower risks and improved tolerability, such as lamotrigine, indicated for prevention of depression in maintenance of bipolar disorder, are sometimes effective; however, others, such as gabapentin, have demonstrated no benefit in prospective trials. Mood stabilizers are a mainstay of treatment; monotherapy with antidepressants in bipolar disorder can precipitate mania.[9] In fact, evidence for the effectiveness of antidepressants in bipolar depression is mixed,[10] and many studies suggest that these drugs are not effective. Thus, it may be prudent to avoid antidepressants as much as possible.

Monitoring is important not only for symptoms of bipolar disorder but also for possible adverse effects of the medications used to treat it. Patients taking lithium require baseline and periodic monitoring of thyroid function, renal function, and white blood cell count. Patients taking valproic acid require baseline and periodic monitoring of hepatic function and platelet count and are at increased risk for the development of pancreatitis. Carbamazepine has been associated with agranulocytosis and hyponatremia, so a metabolic profile and complete blood count should be checked prior to initiating therapy with carbamazepine.

Lamotrigine can be an effective agent, but due to the potential for development of toxic epidermal necrolysis, it cannot be rapidly up-titrated.

A number of atypical antipsychotic medications have been studied and approved for use in acute and maintenance treatment of bipolar disorder. Though they may not require the same drug level monitoring and may have fewer drug–drug interactions than traditional mood stabilizers, patients taking atypical antipsychotic agents require baseline and periodic monitoring of body mass index, abdominal circumference, fasting lipids, and fasting glucose due to their association with the development of obesity, diabetes mellitus, and the metabolic syndrome.[11] Even if regular psychiatric follow-up is impractical, at least consultative input from a psychiatrist is recommended in the management of patients with bipolar disorder.

Table 4.2 Medications used to treat bipolar disorder

Drug name	Usual starting dose1	Effective daily dose range
Lithium[2]	300 to 600 mg at bedtime or bid	Varies; 1200 to 1800 mg Do not exceed 2400 mg daily 0.6 to 0.8 mg/dL serum concentration
Anticonvulsants		
Carbamazepine[3]	200 mg bid	600 to 1200 mg (divided bid) 8 to 12 mg/dL safe serum concentration
Lamotrigine[4]	25 mg once daily	200 mg
Valproic acid[5]	500 to 750 mg, divided bid	1500 to 3000 mg (divided bid) Do not exceed 60 mg/kg daily.
Antipsychotics[6]		
Aripiprazole[7]	15 to 30 mg once daily	15 to 30 mg
Olanzapine	10 to 15 mg at bedtime	20 mg
Quetiapine[8]	50 mg at bedtime	300 mg
Risperidone	1 to 2 mg once daily	2 to 4 mg
Ziprasidone	40 mg bid with food	60 to 80 mg (divided bid)
Other		
Olanzapine[6]/Fluoxetine 6 mg/25 mg once daily		6 to 12/25 to 50 mg

Source: Clinical Pharmacology Online. Available at: http://cpip.gsm.com/.

[1] In nonemergent settings, starting at lower doses may improve tolerability and enhance adherence to the regimen. Use the lowest effective dose in all cases. Patients who appear to be manic should be referred for psychiatric evaluation and possible admission for stability.

[2] Narrow therapeutic index; toxic in overdose. Therapeutic level 0.6 to 0.8; higher levels may be needed in cases of acute mania, and consultation with psychiatrist may be beneficial. Can cause AV nodal block. Do not use in combination with diuretics, NSAIDs, ACE inhibitors, or medications that impair renal function. Obtain a baseline ECG. Monitor thyroid function, complete blood count, renal function at initiation and every 3 to 6 months thereafter. Check a lithium level with routine monitoring and any time symptoms of possible toxicity (dizziness, tremor, confusion, ataxia) develop. Association with Ebstein's anomaly, a cardiac defect, in fetuses exposed to lithium; data are retrospective, and lithium is considered safer than anticonvulsants in bipolar disorder.

[3] Tricyclic structure. No established therapeutic level in bipolar disorder; 8 to 12 in seizure disorder. Incidence of agranulocytosis, possible development of syndrome of inappropriate antidiuretic hormone (SIADH) with hyponatremia. Obtain a baseline ECG; AV block may occur. Monitor basic metabolic panel, liver enzymes, and complete blood count at initiation and periodically thereafter. Teratogenic; not recommended in pregnancy, especially during first trimester.

[4] Initiate at lowest dose; double dose every 2 weeks to 200 mg daily. More rapid titration may lead to development of rash—if this happens, medication must be discontinued due to concerns for Stevens–Johnson syndrome and toxic epidermal necrolysis. Baseline CBC is recommended for monitoring of possible myelosuppressive effects. Potent inducer of cytochrome P450 isoenzyme 3A4; multiple drug–drug interactions possible.

[5] No established therapeutic level in bipolar disorder; 50 to 100 in seizure disorder. Routine monitoring of serum levels not recommended, though it may be helpful in cases of suspected toxicity or nonadherence to medication. Rare reports of fulminant hepatitis, thrombocytopenia; monitor baseline and periodic liver enzymes, ammonia, and complete blood count. Toxicity may include hyperammonemia, which may be improved with L-carnitine therapy. Teratogenic; not recommended in pregnancy, especially during first trimester.

[6] Atypical antipsychotics have been associated with risk for metabolic syndrome; patients should be screened at baseline and periodically for height, weight, body mass index (BMI), fasting lipids, liver enzymes, and fasting glucose level. Baseline ECG and periodic monitoring for prolongation of the QTc interval is recommended. Antipsychotics may cause or exacerbate orthostatic hypotension. Antipsychotics have been associated with movement disorders; screening with a neurological examination and Abnormal Involuntary Movement Scale at baseline and periodically is recommended.

[7] Metabolized by cytochrome P450 isoenzymes 3A4 and 2D6; reduce dose when administered concomitantly with inhibitors, increase dose when administered concomitantly with inducers of these isoenzymes.

[8] Premarketing association with the development of cataracts; baseline ophthalmologic examination and periodic screening are recommended.

Treatment of schizophrenia and chronic psychotic disorders

Table 4.3[1] summarizes medications and doses used in the treatment of schizophrenia. Antipsychotics may also be used to control psychotic symptoms of other illnesses. Most patients with chronic schizophrenia will require prolonged or even indefinite maintenance therapy. Many psychiatrists believe that patients with chronic psychotic disorders are best treated in a multidisciplinary setting with mental health professionals, case management, and vocational rehabilitation (e.g., assertive community treatment or ACT approach).[12] Patients seen in nonpsychiatric settings will sometimes be taking injections of long-acting "depot" formulations of fluphenazine or haloperidol, or the Consta formulation of risperidone. These medications can be associated with movement disorders such as parkinsonism and tardive dyskinesia, as well as other side effects, QTc prolongation, and drug–drug interactions.

The risks of tardive dyskinesia and adverse metabolic effects are concerns with antipsychotic medications, and patients should be treated with the lowest effective dose. Second-generation (atypical) antipsychotics including clozapine, olanzapine, risperidone, quetiapine, ziprasidone, and aripiprazole have not been clearly shown to be more effective or preferable to first-generation (typical) antipsychotics such as perphenazine, though more study is needed.[13] The risk of movement disorders appears to be less with the second-generation (atypical) class. Clozapine is considered the most effective antipsychotic in either class but is also associated with a risk of agranulocytosis and requires weekly complete blood count monitoring.[14] Clozapine has also been associated with myocarditis and seizures and is not considered a first-line agent. Physicians wishing to prescribe clozapine are required to register in the national registry and are obligated to provide systematic weekly complete blood count monitoring and close follow-up; in general, nonpsychiatrists would have no reason to initiate or prescribe ongoing treatment with clozapine. It appears that optimizing the dose of a patient's existing antipsychotic and ensuring adherence to therapy are more effective than switching medications in patients whose symptoms recur.[15]

In addition to routine monitoring of neurological status and screening for the development of abnormal movement disorders, patients prescribed atypical antipsychotics should have baseline and regular monitoring of height, weight, abdominal circumference, fasting lipids, and fasting glucose.[16]

Table 4.3 Medications FDA-approved to treat schizophrenia

Drug name	Usual starting dose[1]	Usual effective daily dose
Second-generation ("atypical") antipsychotics[2]		
Aripiprazole[3]	10 to 15 mg once daily	15 to 30 mg
Olanzapine	5 to 10 mg at bedtime	10 to 20 mg
Paliperidone[4]	6 mg once daily	6 mg (maximum 12 mg)
Quetiapine[5]	50 mg at bedtime	300 mg
Risperidone[6]	1 to 2 mg once or divided bid	4 to 6 mg
Ziprasidone	20 mg twice daily with food	120 to 160 mg (divided bid)
Clozapine[7]	12.5 to 25 mg once or divided bid	300 to 450 mg (divided bid or tid)
First-generation ("typical") antipsychotics[8]		
Chlorpromazine	10 to 25 mg bid to qid	200 to 400 mg (divided bid to qid)
Fluphenazine[9]	2.5 to 10 mg divided bid or tid	15 to 20 mg (divided bid)
Haloperidol[10]	0.5 to 2 mg bid or tid	15 to 20 mg (divided bid or tid)
Loxapine	10 mg bid	60 to 100 mg (once or divided bid)
Molindone	15 to 75 mg divided bid or tid	60 to 100 mg (divided bid or tid)
Perphenazine	12 to 24 mg divided tid	12 to 24 mg (divided bid or tid)
Prochlorperazine	15 to 30 mg divided tid or qid	50 to 100 mg (divided tid or qid)
Thioridazine	10 to 50 mg tid	200 to 300 mg (divided bid to qid)
Thiothixene	6 to 10 mg divided bid or tid	10 to 30 mg (divided bid or tid)
Trifluoperazine	2 to 5 mg once or twice daily	15 to 20 mg (once or divided bid)

Source: Clinical Pharmacology Online. Available at: http://cpip.gsm.com/.

[1] All antipsychotics have been associated with a risk of neuroleptic malignant syndrome, a potentially fatal syndrome involving fever, altered mental status, and hyperreflexia. Antipsychotic treatment has also been associated with QTc prolongation and increased risk for torsades de pointes. Baseline ECG should be obtained before initiating antipsychotic therapy. Other medications may interact with antipsychotic medications. There is a risk of movement disorder with antipsychotic medications, and patients should be monitored at baseline and periodically with the use of the Abnormal Involuntary Movement Scale. The lowest effective dose should be used; after effective antipsychosis has been achieved, work to decrease the dose to the lowest effective dose.

[2] Second-generation antipsychotics have been associated with the development of metabolic syndrome, including weight gain and diabetes mellitus, as well as lipid derangements. Consensus guidelines recommend the following for patients taking atypical antipsychotic medications: Patients should be screened for personal and family history, weight (BMI), waist circumference, blood pressure, fasting glucose, and fasting lipid profile at baseline and 12 weeks, then every 5 years. Weight should be monitored monthly for 3 months and then quarterly after initiating an atypical antipsychotic. Fasting plasma glucose and blood pressure should be monitored at 12 weeks and annually thereafter. Waist circumference should be monitored annually (APA/ADA guidelines. *Diabetes Care.* 2004;27:596–601). Patients should also undergo baseline and periodic screening with the Abnormal Involuntary Movement Scale to document the development of any abnormal movements that might be related to the antipsychotic. There is a boxed warning for atypical antipsychotics addressing the increased mortality in elderly patients with dementia-related psychosis (an off-label use).

[3] Metabolized by cytochrome P450 isoenzymes 3A4 and 2D6; reduce dose when administered concomitantly with inhibitors, increase dose when administered concomitantly with inducers of these isoenzymes.

[4] Less likely to have hepatic cytochrome P450–mediated interactions with other medications. Like risperidone, paliperidone is associated with hyperprolactinemia.

[5] Premarketing association with the development of cataracts; baseline ophthalmologic examination and periodic screening are recommended.

[6] Like paliperidone, risperidone is associated with hyperprolactinemia. Doses higher than 6 mg daily may be associated with a higher incidence of extrapyramidal side effects. Risperidone is available in a long-acting injectable formulation.

[7] In cases of refractory schizophrenia or other disorders requiring clozapine, a psychiatrist should be involved. Clozapine carries boxed warnings about agranulocytosis, seizure risk, myocarditis,

orthostatic hypotension and collapse when used in conjunction with benzodiazepines, and increased mortality in elderly patients with dementia-related psychosis. Clozapine may be prescribed only by physicians who have registered to prescribe it in systems prepared to monitor weekly complete blood count (with manual differential) and provide close follow-up. It is important to avoid benzodiazepines in patients who are taking clozapine.

[8] In addition to baseline ECG and neurological evaluation, many of the first-generation antipsychotics also include recommendations to monitor ophthalmologic examinations, complete blood counts, thyroid function tests, and serum prolactin levels at baseline and periodically.

[9] Fluphenazine is available in a long-acting injectable formulation.

[10] Haloperidol is available in a long-acting injectable formulation.

Treatment of dementia

The development of dementia or progressive cognitive impairment can be distressing to patients, families, and physicians. After underlying reversible etiologies such as thyroid derangements, B_{12} deficiency, neurosyphilis, and other nutritional deficiencies have been ruled out or addressed, cognitive and behavioral issues can still be difficult to manage (refer to Chapter 13, "The Patient with Confusion or Memory Problems," and Chapter 17, "The Geriatric Patient"). Treatment options are limited, and FDA-approved therapies (listed in Table 4.4[1]) are targeted at maximizing independence and functioning by slowing the relentless progression of dementing illness. In cases of vascular dementia, it is important to optimize reduction of vascular risk factors and enhance healthy behaviors. Addition of acetylcholinesterase inhibitors may be helpful. The clinical relevance of improvements seen with cholinesterase inhibitors is debatable, but some patients who tolerate the medications well may derive benefit from them. Side effects including bradycardia and adverse gastrointestinal effects, as well as cost issues, limit their tolerability in some elderly adults.

Although many medications have been tried in the treatment of behavioral disturbances in dementia, the evidence for the effectiveness of most agents, including antipsychotics (which carry a boxed warning regarding the off-label use in dementia and the increased risk of mortality in this population), suggests that there are still no optimal medications for the treatment of dementia and its behavioral disturbances.[17] Some physicians believe that early initiation of a cholinesterase inhibitor with or without the NMDA agonist memantine will provide the best chance for functional preservation in elderly adults suffering from dementia.[18]

In elderly demented patients, it is important to avoid therapies that may worsen cognition, including anticholinergic medications (e.g., diphenhydramine, opiates) and benzodiazepines and their derivatives.

Treatment of disordered sleep/insomnia

When addressing sleep disorders, it is important to rule out underlying medical or psychiatric pathology that would be amenable to treatment with, for example, an antidepressant or mood-stabilizing agent. Nonpharmacological interventions including sleep hygiene and dietary

Table 4.4 Medications used to treat dementia

Drug name	Usual starting dose[1,2]	Usual effective daily dose
Acetylcholinesterase inhibitors[3]		
Donepezil	5 mg once daily	10 mg
Galantamine	4 mg bid with food	16 mg divided bid
Rivastigmine	1.5 mg bid with food	4 to 12 mg divided bid
Transdermal form	4.6 mg/24 hours	4.6 to 9.5 mg/24 hours
Tacrine[4]	10 mg qid	80 mg divided qid
Other medications		
Memantine	5 mg once daily	20 mg divided bid
Ergot mesylates[5]	1 mg tid	3 to 6 mg divided tid

Source: Clinical Pharmacology Online. Available at: http://cpip.gsm.com/.

[1] Antipsychotics have not been approved for use in patients with dementia and agitation. A boxed warning highlights increased mortality risk with antipsychotics and demented elderly patients.

[2] Though not approved, many patients may use over-the-counter remedies such as gingko biloba or SAMe for memory deficits. It is important to screen for the use of these remedies, which may interact with other medications. Gingko biloba is associated with platelet inhibition and may contribute to bleeding risk in patients on other platelet inhibitors, including aspirin, clopidogrel, and SSRIs.

[3] Peripheral nervous system effects of cholinesterase inhibitors can include bradycardia, abdominal discomfort, and GI complaints. Medications with less peripheral nervous system activity (e.g., donepezil) are better tolerated than their older counterparts (e.g., tacrine).

[4] Monitor liver enzymes at baseline and then every 2 weeks for 3 months; if stable, monitor liver enzymes every 3 months.

[5] Though FDA-approved for use in dementia, the American Academy of Neurology recommends further study for efficacy.

measures are important in the development of healthy sleeping patterns. However, a significant number of patients in primary care will request sleep aids (refer to Chapter 15, "The Patient with Disordered Sleep").

Table 4.5[1] summarizes agents that have been approved by the FDA for treatment of insomnia. Most medications are recommended for use in the short term; only eszopiclone has been approved for longer-term use. In general, side effects of sedative/hypnotic medications include cognitive impairment, day-after drowsiness, and risk of dependence. Of note, though trazodone is frequently used in cases of insomnia, it is not approved as a sleep aid, and there is limited evidence supporting its use for this purpose.[19] Older medications, including barbiturates and other agents such as chloral hydrate, are not considered acceptable sleep aids and should be carefully tapered and discontinued whenever possible. The use of sleep aids in long-term care facilities is federally regulated, and dosage and duration limits apply.

Treatment of substance abuse

Treatment of substance abuse or dependence frequently requires non-pharmacologic interventions (cognitive-behavioral therapy, 12-step groups, reinforcement) as well as consideration of appropriate pharmacotherapy (refer to Chapter 10, "The Patient with Disordered Use of Substances or Alcohol"). Formal input from an addictions specialist may be beneficial or

Table 4.5 Medications used to treat insomnia

Drug name	Usual dose[1]	Comments
Melatonin receptor agonist		
Ramelteon[2]	8 mg at bedtime	
Non-benzodiazepine GABAA receptor agonists		
Eszopiclone	1 to 2 mg at bedtime	Maximum dose 3 mg
Zaleplon	5 to 10 mg at bedtime	Maximum dose 20 mg
Zolpidem	5 to 10 mg at bedtime	Do not exceed 10 mg/day.
Histamine H1 Receptor Blockers[3]		
Acetaminophen + diphenhydramine	Variable per formulation 500 mg APAP/12.5 to 50 mg diphenhydramine	
Diphenhydramine	25 to 50 mg at bedtime	
Doxylamine	25 mg at bedtime	For <2 weeks' use
Benzodiazepines[4]		
Estazolam	1 to 2 mg at bedtime	
Flurazepam	15 mg at bedtime	Maximum dose 30 mg
Quazepam	7.5 to 15 mg at bedtime	
Temazepam	7.5 to 15 mg at bedtime	Maximum dose 30 mg
Barbiturates[5]		
Aprobarbital	40 to 160 mg at bedtime	
Butabarbital	50 to 100 mg at bedtime	
Pentobarbital	100 to 200 mg at bedtime	
Secobarbital[6]	100 to 200 mg at bedtime	
Other agents[7]		
Chloral hydrate[8]	500 to 1000 mg at bedtime	
Ethchlorvynol[9]	500 to 1000 mg at bedtime	
Paraldehyde[10]	4 to 8 mg at bedtime	

Source: Clinical Pharmacology Online. Available at: http://cpip.gsm.com/.

[1] The FDA requires information including the following to be provided to patients with each prescription and refill of sedative–hypnotic medications: *Sedative–hypnotic medications have been associated with behaviors including sleep-driving, making phone calls, or eating while asleep.* Most sleep aids have been approved or recommended only for short-term (e.g., less than 14 days) use. Patients should be advised not to drive or participate in dangerous activities after taking the medications and even the next day. All but one prescription sedative–hypnotic medications are controlled substances.

[2] Ramelteon is the first prescription sedative–hypnotic approved as a noncontrolled substance. Patients should be counseled to avoid eating a high-fat meal in proximity to ramelteon. Significant drug–drug interactions through CYP450 1A2 isoenzyme are possible.

[3] Anticholinergic medications can cause cognitive impairment, delirium, and next-day drowsiness.

[4] Elderly patients have delayed clearance of benzodiazepines and should be prescribed the lowest possible dose (frequently half the usual starting dose). Side effects include possible cognitive impairment, respiratory depression, and next-day drowsiness.

[5] Barbiturates are no longer considered acceptable sleep aids. If patients are taking these medications, it is important to taper carefully and discontinue. Barbiturates lose effectiveness after 14 days and are restricted by federal guidelines in institutionalized patients. Adverse liver effects, teratogenicity, Stevens-Johnson syndrome, respiratory depression, and potential drug–drug interactions are all possible.

[6] Secobarbital, while approved for insomnia, is not accepted as a safe sleep aid.

[7] There is no good reason to use any of these medications, which have generally been replaced by newer, safer sedative–hypnotics. Patients should not take these medications for more than 7 to 14 days; if a patient is taking one of these medications long term, it is a good idea to taper carefully and discontinue.

[8] Chloral hydrate is contraindicated in hepatic or renal impairment.

[9] Ethchlorvynol is not recommended for more than 7 days' use; contraindicated in porphyria and hepatic or renal impairment and has high dependence potential.

[10] Paraldehyde has high potential for physical dependence. It is contraindicated in bronchopulmonary disorders, hepatic impairment, or gastrointestinal disorders. Concomitant administration of disulfiram should be avoided.

Table 4.6 Medications used to treat alcohol and drug dependence

Drug name	Usual starting dose	Usual effective daily dose[1]
Drugs for alcohol dependence		
Acamprosate[7]	666 mg tid	1332 to 1998 mg (divided bid or tid)
Disulfiram[3]	500 mg once daily	125 to 500 mg
Naltrexone[4]	50 mg once daily with food	50 to 100 mg
Drugs for opiate dependence		
Buprenorphine[5]	8 mg once daily (sublingual)	16 mg (maximum 24 mg)
Methadone[6]	20 to 40 mg once daily	Varies (maximum 120 mg)
Naltrexone[7]	25 mg once daily	50 to 150 mg once or divided
Drugs for nicotine dependence		
Bupropion[8]	150 mg once daily	300 mg divided bid
Nicotine		
Lozenges[9]	2 to 4 mg every 1 to 2 hours	2 to 4 mg, taper after 6 weeks
Chewing gum[10]	2 mg with any urge to smoke	20 mg (maximum 60)
Transdermal[11]	14 to 21 mg/24 hours[8]	Varies (maximum 22 mg/24 hours)
Varenicline[12]	0.5 mg once daily	2 mg divided bid

Source: Clinical Pharmacology Online. Available at: http://cpip.gsm.com/.

[1] Psychosocial counseling and/or psychotherapy are crucial components of any treatment plan that includes pharmacotherapy for alcohol and drug dependence.

[2] Acamprosate is contraindicated in renal impairment (CrCl < 30 mg/min).

[3] Disulfiram is contraindicated in patients with cardiac disease (history of myocardial infarction or coronary occlusive disease), alcohol intoxication, or psychosis. Patients and families should be informed of adverse reactions that occur when alcohol-containing substances are consumed and should carry an emergency card describing such reactions. Disulfiram should never be prescribed to a patient who is unaware of the risks and potential adverse effects. Liver enzymes should be monitored every 10 to 14 days and complete blood count and electrolytes should be checked at baseline and every 6 months during disulfiram therapy.

[4] Liver enzymes should be monitored in patients undergoing naltrexone therapy, and naltrexone should not be given to patients with hepatic impairment or hepatic encephalopathy. Do not give naltrexone to patients with ongoing substance abuse, and hold the medication for 7 days prior to any anesthesia-requiring procedures.

[5] Physicians must meet certain criteria to prescribe buprenorphine. Physicians prescribing buprenorphine can prescribe the drug to only 30 patients at one time.

[6] Methadone may be prescribed only in accordance with Federal Methadone Regulations and prescribed and dispensed by pharmacies and treatment facilities meeting these regulations as assessed by FDA and state regulatory agencies. Doses above 120 mg in the clinic or 100 mg at home require prior approval by the FDA and state agencies. Methadone maintenance can be ongoing for years in some patients and must be accomplished through an accredited methadone maintenance program with an addiction specialist prescribing the medication. Patients claiming a daily dose of methadone through a maintenance program need to provide the contact information for the program, and the nonpsychiatric physician is obligated to verify the daily dose and enrollment in the program before prescribing an equivalent dose in the nonpsychiatric setting (e.g., medical–surgical setting).

[7] Naltrexone is FDA-designated an orphan drug for opiate dependence. Liver enzymes should be monitored in patients undergoing naltrexone therapy, and naltrexone should not be given to patients with hepatic impairment or hepatic encephalopathy. Do not give naltrexone to patients with ongoing substance abuse, and hold the medication for 7 days prior to any anesthesia-requiring procedures.

[8] Treatment with bupropion should begin 1 to 2 weeks prior to the "quit date" set by the patient. Bupropion lowers the seizure threshold and should not be used in patients with a history of seizures, head trauma, or electrolyte abnormalities that predispose to seizures.

[9] Nicotine lozenges should be dosed depending on "time to first cigarette"—2 mg if first morning cigarette is smoked >30 minutes after awakening, 4 mg if first morning cigarette is smoked <30 minutes after awakening. Stable dose for 6 weeks, then taper; duration of use should not exceed 12 weeks.

[10] Nicotine gum should not be continued for more than 3 months. In trials, 2 mg dose did not separate from placebo; 4 mg dose was effective. Dose should not exceed 60 mg daily, and duration should not exceed 6 months.

[11] Nicotine patch dosage depends on weight, cardiovascular morbidity, and number of cigarettes per day. There are different formulations and dosages (21/14/7 mg/24 hours, 15/10/5 mg/24 hours, and 22/11 mg/24 hours). If weight is greater than 100 lb, the patient smokes at least one pack of cigarettes daily, and cardiovascular disease is absent, the higher dose is appropriate. In patients who weigh less than 100 lbs, smoke less than one pack per day, or have cardiovascular disease, the middle dose is appropriate. In all cases, daily dose should be tapered every 2 to 4 weeks with a goal of discontinuation by the end of 8 weeks.

[12] Duration of varenicline for successful quit attempt may extend to 24 weeks; patients who are unsuccessful after a 12-week trial should discontinue the medication and try again after factors contributing to failed quit attempt are addressed.

even required for the provision of pharmacotherapy. Only specially licensed providers, pharmacies, and treatment facilities can prescribe methadone and buprenorphine, and such use is subject to regulation by the FDA, DEA, and state regulatory agencies. Patients who claim to be taking methadone maintenance for opiate dependence may require methadone in medical or surgical (e.g., inpatient) settings, but the physician must verify the dose and ongoing enrollment in treatment with the accredited facility before prescribing the amount claimed by the patient. Table 4.6[1] summarizes medications approved for the treatment of alcohol and drug abuse. Use of these medications without nonpharmacological intervention for substance abuse is not advised.

References

1. Clinical Pharmacology Online. Available at: http://cpip.gsm.com/. Accessed October 22–24, 2007.

2. General principles of psychopharmacological treatment. In: Schatzberg AF, Cole JO, DeBattista C, eds. Manual of Clinical Psychopharmacology, 6th ed. Arlington, VA: American Psychiatric Publishing, Inc.; 2007.

3. Cytochrome P450 system: Drug interactions. Abbreviated clinical table. Indiana University School of Medicine Web site. Available at: http://medicine.iupui.edu/flockhart/clinlist.htm. Accessed October 26, 2007.

4. Ward RK, Zamorski MA. Benefits and risks of psychiatric medications during pregnancy. Am Fam Phys. 2002;66:629–636.

5. Drugs for psychiatric disorders. Med Lett Treatment Guidelines. 2006;4(46):35–46.

6. American Psychiatric Association. Practice Guideline for the Treatment of Patients with Major Depressive Disorder, 2nd ed. Available at: http://www.psych.org/psych_pract/treatg/pg/MDD2e_05–15–06.pdf. Accessed September 26, 2007.

7. Fancher T, Kravitz R. In the clinic: depression. Ann Intern Med. 2007; 146:ITC5–1.

8. Carvalho AF, Cavalcante JL, Castelo MS, Lima MC. Augmentation strate- gies for treatment-resistant depression: a literature review. *J Clin Pharm Ther.* 2007;32:415–428.

9. McIntosh A, Cohen A, Turnbull N, et al. *Clinical Guidelines for the Management of Anxiety. Management of Anxiety (Panic Disorder, with or without Agoraphobia, and Generalised Anxiety Disorder) in Adults in Primary, Secondary and Community Care.* London: National Institute for Clinical Excellence (NICE); 2004. Available at: http://www.guideline.gov/summary/summary.aspx?doc_id=6248. Accessed November 28, 2007.

10. Lin D, Mok H, Lakshmi N. Polytherapy in bipolar disorder: therapy in practice. *CNS Drugs.* 2006;20:29–42.

11. Belmaker RH. Treatment of bipolar depression. *N Engl J Med.* 2007;10.1056/ NEJMc078042.

12. American Diabetes Association, American Psychiatric Association, American Association of Clinical Endocrinologists, North American Association for the Study of Obesity. Consensus development conference on antipsychotic drugs and obesity and diabetes. *Diabetes Care.* 2004;27:596–601.

13. Marshall M, Rathbone J. Early intervention for psychosis. *Cochrane Database of Systematic Reviews.* 2006, Issue 4. Art. No.: CD004718. DOI: 10.1002/14651858. CD004718.pub2.

14. Lieberman JA, Stroup TS, McEvoy JP, et al. Effectiveness of antipsychotic drugs in patients with chronic schizophrenia. *N Engl J Med.* 2005;353:1209–1223.

15. Hennen J, Baldessarini RJ. Suicidal risk during treatment with clozapine: a meta- analysis. *Schizophr Res.* 2005;73:139–145.

16. Essock SM, Covell NH, Davis SM, Stroup TS, Rosenheck RA, Lieberman JA. Effectiveness of switching antipsychotic medications. *Am J Psychiatry.* 2006;163:2090–2095.

17. Sink KM, Holden KF, Yaffe K. Pharmacological treatment of neuropsychiatric symptoms of dementia: a review of the evidence. *JAMA.* 2005;293:596–608.

18. Geldmacher DS. Treatment guidelines for Alzheimer's disease: redefin- ing perceptions in primary care. *Prim Care Companion J Clin Psychiatry.* 2007; 9:113–121.

19. Mendelson WB. A review of the evidence for the efficacy and safety of trazodone in insomnia. *J Clin Psychiatry.* 2005;66:469–476.

Chapter 5

Psychiatric emergencies

Y. Pritham Raj

To write this chapter, several resident physicians who stand at the front lines of patient care were asked for an overview of their experiences with the psychiatric emergencies that they most frequently encounter but feel least prepared to handle. The following list, not structured in order of importance, targets the highlights. Most are discussed in greater detail in other chapters of this text.

Clinical Scenario 1

DP is a 59-year-old divorced car salesman (currently between jobs) who has been followed in the outpatient clinic for more than 3 years. Medically, he has a history of stage I hypertension, hyperlipidemia, and impaired glucose tolerance—all generally controlled with a combination of diet, exercise, hydrochlorothiazide, and atorvastatin. Mr. P has also been treated for major depression with a selective serotonin reuptake inhibitor (SSRI). He was psychiatrically hospitalized once in the last year for suicidal ideation and was discharged after 3 days. As part of his ongoing primary care, Dr. Y periodically monitors his symptoms with the Patient Hospital Questionnaire-9 (PHQ-9) (refer to Chapter 7, "The Patient with Depressive Symptoms"). Today, Mr. P's score has doubled from 10 at last visit to 20. He appears more despondent and hopeless as a result of his continued inability to find work. He is also rather restless. He mentions having intermittent suicidal thoughts, though when he is asked he denies having active plans for killing himself at the moment.

What is the best course of action?

Suicidality

Mood deterioration to the point of suicidality is one of the most commonly encountered psychiatric emergencies in the outpatient setting, with a 2% to 3% prevalence rate in the United States among primary care patients.[1] Acording to U.S. Centers for Disease Control data,[2] a staggering 89 Americans take their own lives daily, rendering suicide the 11th leading cause of death in the United States. But only a little over one-third of physicians treating depressed patients assess for suicide (this subject is discussed in more detail in Chapter 6, "Suicide Risk Assessment"). The importance of systematic safety screening cannot be overemphasized. The system outlined in Table 5.1[3] is a helpful tool for the *reasonable* assessment of safety

Table 5.1 Features of a systematic suicide assessment
• Ask gently whether suicidal thoughts are still present (reviewing protective factors may also be helpful—responsibility to family, moral objections, etc.).
• Assess for delirium—the Folstein Mini-Mental State Exam (MMSE)[4] or Mini-cog can be helpful as a snapshot in cognitive assessment.
• Assess for psychosis—screening for auditory or visual hallucinations is generally sufficient.
• Assess for depression (as discussed in Chapter 7).
• Quote what the patient plans to do for follow-up—perhaps offer a suggestion if needed. Referral to a mental health provider may be indicated here.
• Collateral from and discussion with a third party—this is an underused but often useful step where the patient's family member or confidant is present during the discussion of the aftercare plan.

Reprinted from Goldberg RJ. Assessment of suicide risk in the general hospital. *General Hospital Psychiatry*. 1987;9:446–452, with permission from Elsevier.

(the legal standard) when deciding whether outpatients are safe to leave the office or inpatients who have reported suicidal thoughts are safe for discharge. A provider can document all of the elements listed below in a few simple sentences, with no more than a few minutes required to complete the entire assessment.

Serotonin syndrome

This emergency must also be considered in any patient taking serotonergic medication who appears restless. As the triad of mental status changes, autonomic hyperactivity, and neuromuscular abnormalities, serotonin syndrome is actually a spectrum of clinical findings ranging from benign to lethal; the intensity of clinical findings is thought to reflect the degree of serotonergic activity. Common presentations include agitated delirium, restlessness, disorientation, easy startling, diaphoresis, tachycardia, hyperthermia, hypertension, vomiting, tremor, muscle rigidity, myoclonus, hyperreflexia, and bilateral Babinski sign. Serotonin syndrome can be easily mistaken for anxiety or agitation. This often leads to an erroneous dose escalation in serotonergic medication by the prescribing physician, which worsens symptoms. Drug interactions are perhaps the most common cause of serotonin syndrome, which also needs to be differentiated from neuroleptic malignant syndrome, anticholinergic toxicity, malignant hyperthermia, and sympathomimetic toxicity.

The following actions are essential in the management of serotonin syndrome, although their application varies with the severity of illness:

- Discontinue all serotonergic agents.
- Provide supportive care aiming at normalization of vital signs, selecting a short-acting antihypertensive agent when it is needed.
- Use benzodiazepines judiciously for sedation in the agitated patient.
- Consider administering a serotonin antidote—cyproheptadine is the antidote with the best proven efficacy.[4]
- Assess the need to resume use of causative serotonergic agents after resolution of symptoms.

Serotonin syndrome often resolves within 24 hours of discontinuing the serotonergic agent, but drugs with long half-lives or active metabolites may cause symptoms to persist.[5]

Clinical scenario 2

Mr. P returns to the office 10 days after his most recent visit. Since his last visit he has seen a psychiatrist, who augmented his SSRI with lithium, which he started 5 days ago. He says he now feels a bit restless and shaky but no longer feels suicidal. Remembering that there are several classes of common medications that should be used with absolute caution (if at all) with lithium (ACE inhibitors, angiotensin receptor blockers, NSAIDs, and diuretics [thiazides worse than loop]), Dr. Y decides to stop Mr. P's hydrochlorothiazide and check a lithium level.

Are there other labs that should be monitored?

Lithium toxicity

This elemental salt, seen on the periodic table right above sodium, is traditionally used as a mood stabilizer to treat bipolar disorder but has received attention as an augmentation strategy for depression (refer to Chapter 4, "Overview of Psychopharmacologic Therapies"). It has shown an ability to reduce the rate of suicide. Lithium toxicity is encountered frequently and must be understood. In most cases, psychiatrists should take the lead as primary prescribers/monitors of lithium. Generally, a circulating lithium level should be checked every 3 to 6 months or after 5 to 7 days of any dose adjustment, obtained as a trough level (i.e., 12 hours after the last dose). However, any time a patient on lithium reports symptoms of blurred vision, increased GI disturbances, muscle weakness, drowsiness and sluggishness, ataxia, coarse tremor, lack of coordination, dysarthria, confusion, or convulsions, a lithium level must be checked immediately and consideration should be given to holding lithium, as lithium toxicity is a medical and psychiatric emergency.

Ten thousand cases of lithium toxicity occur annually in the United States alone—a statistic that is on the rise. The traditional therapeutic range for lithium is between 0.4 and 1.1 mEq/L. However, deaths have been reported at even safe/therapeutic lithium levels, rendering the clinical picture essential to any assessment of lithium toxicity. Most guidelines[6] recommend monitoring thyroid and renal function at least annually. The latter is checked via the serum creatinine, with most laboratories now calculating an estimation of the glomerular filtration rate. One approach is to check the serum creatinine whenever checking a lithium level—particularly in elderly patients or those who have multiple medical problems and/or take multiple medications—because patients who initially presented within a "safe" lithium range but had undiagnosed deterioration in renal function are at high risk for lithium toxicity that, if detected sooner, could have been prevented. Other electrolytes, blood urea, urine protein, vital signs (including blood pressure and weight), and even electrocardiograms in the elderly have been recommended for routine monitoring on lithium.

Treatment of lithium toxicity depends on the adequacy of renal function and the degree of intoxication. In addition to discontinuing lithium, fluid repletion, reduction of intestinal absorption, and hemodialysis may be necessary when the lithium level is above 4 mEq/L or above 2.5 mEq/L in patients who are markedly symptomatic or have renal insufficiency or other conditions that can limit urinary lithium excretion (such as congestive heart failure or cirrhosis).[7]

Clinical Scenario 3

At last evaluation, Mr. P was discovered to have only a mild lithium elevation. Hemodialysis was never considered given that his renal function was good and he stabilized clinically with a simple dose reduction. Today, he presents with a productive cough, fever to 38.5°C, and general malaise. He admits that financial stress has been mounting and that he has been drinking more alcohol than usual. He has drunk heavily in the past, but it never impaired his functioning. Chest radiograph confirms lobar pneumonia, and Dr. Y decides to admit Mr. P to the hospital because of a systolic blood pressure hovering at 90 mmHg as part of a dehydration picture. In the hospital he grows agitated and confused.

Alcohol withdrawal

The main concern in patients with alcohol abuse or dependence is the development of delirium tremens (DTs), which occurs in about 5% of withdrawal states but carries up to a 35% mortality rate if left untreated. The mortality figure drops below 5% when adequate treatment is in place. Benzodiazepines are the best prophylaxis and/or treatment for potential DTs and other alcohol withdrawal states. As monotherapy, benzodiazepines are recommended with substantial clinical confidence in most practice guidelines.[8] However, a Cochrane analysis recently found no major difference in effect between the benzodiazepines and anticonvulsants such as carbamazepine and valproic acid in the treatment of alcohol withdrawal.[9] More data are needed before definitive conclusions can be drawn from this comparison.

When treating with benzodiazepines, the drug of choice for a patient with normal hepatic function is chlordiazepoxide, as it is long-acting and easy to taper. Lorazepam is a good choice when there are concerns about liver impairment. A scheduled drug dosing regimen is generally the safest strategy in hospitals with routine nursing care and should be used as part of a slow taper, with usually no more than a 10% reduction in dose per day. If a hospital unit is able to provide vigilant monitoring of a patient's withdrawal symptoms (at least hourly), a validated protocol using the Clinical Institute Withdrawal Assessment for Alcohol Scale, Revised (CIWA-Ar) could be considered using symptom-triggered benzodiazepine dosing.[10] Great caution must be exercised as this protocol was best validated in dedicated drug detoxification centers with uncomplicated patients and skilled evaluators. (Refer to Chapter 10, "The Patient with Disordered Use of Substances and Alcohol," and Chapter 4, "Overview of Psychopharmacologic Therapies").

Delirium

Apart from concerns about alcohol withdrawal, the clinical situation described above paints a strong picture of delirium, the most commonly encountered inpatient psychiatric emergency. The diagnosis can be made using the "Four C's," which summarize the DSM-IV[11] criteria:

Consciousness—disturbed with reduced ability to focus, sustain, or shift attention

Cognition—changed (memory, orientation, or language) or a perceptual disturbance that is not better accounted for by a dementia

Course—develops over a short period of time (usually hours to days) and waxes/wanes

Consequence—of a general medical condition

The primary prevention of delirium should be the goal of every hospital unit everywhere, given that delirium is associated with a 12-month mortality rate of nearly 40%. Perhaps the best way to prevent delirium is via standardized hospital protocols that protect the most basic sensory and neurovegetative needs of inpatients such as sleep, mobility, vision, hearing, and hydration status.[12]

There are myriad causes of delirium, and the causes should be sought in order to stop delirium. Some causes require urgent attention, including drug withdrawal or Wernicke's encephalopathy; hypoxemia; hypoperfusion (including from acute myocardial infarction, sepsis, etc.); hypertensive encephalopathy; intracranial bleeding; meningitis or encephalitis; and poisons/toxic medication ingestion (refer to Chapter 13, "The Patient with Confusion and Memory Problems," and Chapter 11, "The Patient with Agitated Symptoms"). An easy way to remember the key elements of the acute management of delirium is outlined in Table 5.2 using the Stop, Drop, and ROLL mnemonic—borrowing from the National Fire Protection Association's campaign on what to do if one catches fire. It is appropriate

---

Table 5.2 Acute management of delirium: Stop, drop, and ROLL

- Stop and perform the ABCs of lifesaving—assessing airway, breathing, and circulation; obtain an arterial blood gas if respiratory distress is noted.
- Drop any offending medications/drugs such as anticholinergics. Administer any antidotes if needed (e.g., physostigmine, flumazenil, naloxone).
- R—Radiology (selectively), such as chest radiograph and head CT if risk factors are present for bleeding, trauma, etc.
- O—Organize a safety plan with nursing to include bed rails and sitter if required.
- L—Laboratory studies (complete metabolic set, thyroid-stimulating hormone, folate, B$_{12}$, and RPR), including fever workup as needed.
- L—Loved ones must be mobilized for collateral information and to provide familiar faces to the patient. Plus, it is good form to apprise families that delirium is present.

because there are few "fires" bigger in inpatient medicine than dealing with the agitated, delirious patient.

The treatment of delirium is tied to the determination and treatment of the *underlying* cause (refer to Chapter 13, "The Patient with Confusion or Memory Problems," and Chapter 11, "The Patient with Agitated Symptoms"). The role of antipsychotics in treating delirium is largely extrapolated from studies in dementia and psychosis and is complicated by a boxed warning indicating increased mortality in that setting as well as lack of indication for antipsychotics in delirium (refer to Chapter 4, "Overview of Psychopharmacologic Therapies"). Psychiatric consultation is often beneficial when antipsychotics are being considered for the delirious patient (refer to Chapter 2, "When to Call for Psychiatric Help").

Violence/agitation

Patients who begin to exhibit violent or agitated behavior, most often the result of psychosis, delirium, or even dementia, pose a danger to themselves and others and must be treated without delay. Along with behavioral redirection, early pharmacotherapy, typically with antipsychotics, is among the best initial interventions to prevent the agitated patient's condition from escalating. Offering early pharmacotherapy is also consistent with the principles of patient-centered medicine. Every effort must be made to avoid physical restraints, but when the agitated or violent patient's behavior has become exceedingly dangerous and cannot be controlled by other means, the use of restraints may be appropriate. A familiarity with federal and institutional policies on the use of restraints is of great benefit when treating the violent or agitated patient (refer to Chapter 11, "The Patient with Agitated Symptoms").

Clinical scenario 4

Mr. P received haloperidol for agitation in delirium, and his nurse noted a few hours later that he was febrile and somewhat stiff. What is the primary concern?

Neuroleptic malignant syndrome (NMS)

While acute dystonias are a more common adverse effect with acute antipsychotic use, they tend to resolve quickly after discontinuation of the offending medication. However, NMS, which occurs in 0.5% to 2% of patients treated with antipsychotics, is potentially fatal. It can be thought of as a cousin to serotonin syndrome except that it is precipitated by antipsychotics (conventional or atypical) rather than serotonergic medication. It is typically associated with "lead pipe" muscular rigidity, muscle breakdown (elevated creatinine phosphokinase), fever, autonomic dysfunction, and delirium. In many ways it is like a "stiff" version of serotonin syndrome. In addition to serotonin syndrome, malignant catatonia shares clinical features of hyperthermia and rigidity with NMS (refer to Chapter 19, "The Patient with Unusual Presentations"). Certain conditions or illnesses involving the central nervous system may also manifest similarly to NMS, such as central nervous system infection (e.g., meningitis, encephalitis), systemic infections (e.g., pneumonia, sepsis), seizures, acute hydrocephalus, acute spinal cord injury, heat stroke (neuroleptics predispose to heat stroke by impairing thermoregulation), tetanus, central nervous system vasculitis, thyrotoxicosis, acute porphyria, and so forth.

The best treatment for NMS is discontinuing the offending medication and initiating intensive care support and monitoring. Oddly enough, the ICU setting has its own set of intrinsic risks; the environment has been associated with increased symptoms of confusion, depression, and anxiety even within a normal, non-delirious cohort.[13] Several medications have been studied for use in NMS, but no panacea has emerged.

Clinical scenario 5

Mr. P is eventually discharged and does well at home but develops nagging biliary colic. His surgeon would like to perform elective cholecystectomy and seeks preoperative screening. Mr. P's Cardiac Risk Index score is very low, but Dr. Y discusses with him the events of his last hospitalization, including delirium. He asks whether Dr. Y can determine his risk for postoperative delirium.

Postoperative delirium

This is a heterogeneous disorder with multiple risk factors. A validated prediction rule for delirium after elective noncardiac surgery[14] includes several independent risk factors for delirium, including age 70 or older; self-reported alcohol abuse; poor cognitive status; poor functional status; markedly abnormal preoperative serum sodium, potassium, or glucose; noncardiac thoracic surgery; and aortic aneurysm surgery. The risk of delirium is positively correlated with the number of risk factors present. A recent systematic review highlights two risk factors with strongest predictability for the development of postoperative delirium: preoperative cognitive impairment and psychotropic drug use.[15] The management of postoperative delirium is the same as the management of delirium in general.

Clinical scenario 6

Ms. P, Mr. P's 40-year-old younger sister, has a history of depression and fibromyalgia. She presents to the emergency department reporting vague abdominal pain. She avoids eye contact and has a welt on her arm that she appears to be trying to cover up.

Intimate partner violence (IPV) and rape

Expert consensus suggests that physicians should ask patients about IPV whenever it enters the differential diagnosis. IPV generally develops as a slow, chronic process, rarely presenting as a "true emergency." However, prompt recognition and intervention are essential. Asking patients in a nonjudgmental, supportive fashion when they are alone about suspected abuse is most effective.[16] Screening questions that specifically assess for physical or emotional abuse are best. These include questions such as "Has anyone hurt you physically, for example by pushing, hitting, slapping, or kicking you, or forcing you to have sex?" or "Do you feel threatened or controlled by anyone in your life? Is your partner jealous?" Mandatory reporting of IPV by health care professionals to local law enforcement varies from state to state, with only two states (California and Colorado) currently mandating disclosure. It is essential to assess the patient for safety, including suicidal and homicidal ideation.

Rape protocols also vary from state to state. If a patient is suspected of having been raped, especially within the past 72 hours, a special sexual assault evidence kit or rape kit examination is recommended. Many states offer anonymous testing if the victim prefers it. Many hospitals have trained nurses who assist in performing the rape kit and who serve as the liaison with law enforcement, who assist in the subsequent safety assessment.

Other emergencies

Acute psychosis and capacity are covered in other chapters of this text (refer to Chapter 12, "The Patient with Psychotic Symptoms," and Chapter 20, "The Patient who Refuses Care"). For a more comprehensive review of psychiatric emergencies, Kaplan and Sadock's *Synopsis of Psychiatry: Behavioral Sciences/Clinical Psychiatry*, currently in its ninth edition, provides excellent tables and discussion but is written with the trainee in psychiatry and the practicing mental health professional in mind.

Psychiatric aftercare

Patients who have faced any psychiatric emergency often need to be followed up by a mental health professional. This is particularly important for patients with an underlying, primary psychiatric illness or those who have been prescribed psychotropic medications. Community-based psychiatric services are, in general, more effective and provide greater patient satisfaction than hospital-based care.[17] For patients with chronic, disabling psychiatric illness, an outpatient case manager can also be of great benefit.

References

1. Paykel ES, Myers JK, Lindenthal JJ, Tanner J. Suicidal feelings in the general population. A prevalence study. *Br J Psychiatry*. 1974;124:460–469.
2. Suicide Facts at a Glance. Available at: http://www.cdc.gov/ncipc/dvp/suicide/SuicideDataSheet.pdf. Accessed December 31, 2007.
3. Goldberg RJ. The assessment of suicide risk in the general hospital. *Gen Hosp Psychiatry*. 1987;9:446–452.

4. Graudins A, Stearman A, Chan B. Treatment of the serotonin syndrome with cyproheptadine. *J Emerg Med.* 1998;16:615–619.

5. Boyer EW, Shannon M. The serotonin syndrome. *N Engl J Med.* 2005; 352:1112–1120.

6. Nicholson J, Fitzmaurice B. Monitoring patients on lithium—a good practice guideline. *Psychiatric Bull.* 2002;26:348–351.

7. Zimmerman JL. Poisonings and overdoses in the intensive care unit: general and specific management issues. *Crit Care Med.* 2003;31:2794–2801.

8. Practice Guideline for the Treatment of Patients with Delirium. Available at: www.psych.org/psych_pract/treatg/pg/DeliriumPG_05–15–06.pdf. Accessed October 7, 2007.

9. Polycarpou A, Papanikolaou P, Ioannidis JPA, Contopoulos-Ioannidis DG. Anticonvulsants for alcohol withdrawal. *Cochrane Database Syst Rev.* 2005, Issue 3. Art. No.: CD005064. DOI: 10.1002/14651858.CD005064.pub2.

10. Sullivan JT, Sykora K, Schneiderman J, et al. Assessment of alcohol withdrawal: the revised Clinical Institute Withdrawal Assessment for alcohol scale (CIWA-Ar). *Br J Addict.* 1989;84:1353–1357.

11. American Psychiatric Association. *Diagnostic and Statistical Manual of Mental Disorders, 4th ed., Text Revision.* Washington, DC: American Psychiatric Association; 2000.

12. Inouye SK, Bogardus ST, Charpentier PA, et al. A multicomponent intervention to prevent delirium in hospitalized older patients. *N Engl J Med.* 1999;340:669–676.

13. Tanimoto S, Takayanagi K, Yokota H, Yamamoto Y. The psychological and physiological effects of an intensive-care unit environment on healthy individuals. *Clin Perform Qual Health Care.* 1999;72:77–82.

14. Marcantonio ER, Goldman L, Mangione CM, et al. A clinical prediction rule for delirium after elective noncardiac surgery. *JAMA.* 1994;271:134–139.

15. Dasgupta M, Dumbrell AC. Preoperative risk assessment for delirium after noncardiac surgery: a systematic review. *J Am Geriatr Soc.* 2006;54:1578–1589.

16. Nicolaidis C. Intimate partner violence: a practical guide for primary care clinicians. *Women's Health in Primary Care.* 2004;7:349–362.

17. Merson S, Tyrer P, Onyett S, et al. Early intervention in psychiatric emergencies: a controlled clinical trial. *Lancet.* 1992;339(8805):1311–1314.

Chapter 6

Suicide risk assessment

Eric J. Christopher

Clinical Scenario

Mr. R is a 65-year-old man followed in the primary care clinic. He has a history of prostate cancer and previously documented alcohol abuse. He presents for his usual follow-up visit with Dr. G and reports that his health has been about the same. He says his wife died 2 months ago and his children have not spoken with him since he got drunk at the reception following the funeral. He is a Korean War veteran and was married to his wife for 35 years before her recent death from breast cancer. His four grown children live in the area. He has been retired for the past 5 years and spends his time hunting and fishing. Although he admits to drinking a "little bit," he denies significant drinking problems. His physical examination is unremarkable. Dr. G refills his medications and schedules a 6-month follow-up appointment. Two weeks later, Dr. G learns that Mr. R was found dead from a self-inflicted gunshot wound.

Background

Suicide—intentional and self-inflicted death—is a major contributor to mortality worldwide. Suicidal ideation and suicide attempts are psychiatric emergencies. To understand suicide risk, several terms must be defined. Suicidal ideation (SI) is the thought of killing oneself. A suicide attempt is a definitive action to end one's life. Parasuicide is used to describe actions a patient may take that are not intended to cause death. Parasuicides are also considered "near" suicide or "suicidal gestures." Parasuicides tend to be more characteristic of personality disorders such as borderline personality disorder.

In general, patients contemplating suicide may be undergoing a crisis that causes intense suffering, feelings of hopelessness or helplessness, conflicting emotions about survival and intolerable stress, inability to see past a specific situation, or a wish to escape. Elderly Caucasian males lacking social support are at high risk for committing suicide. It is important for nonpsychiatric physicians to assess patients for SI and suicide risk, especially because studies show that most elderly patients who complete suicide were seen by their primary care providers shortly before the event.[1]

Any patient thought to be at risk for suicide should be immediately referred to a psychiatrist (refer to Chapter 2, "When to Call for Psychiatric Help").

Suicide statistics and suicide risks

In 2004, suicide caused 873,000 deaths worldwide and was the 13th leading cause of death. In the United States, it was the 11th leading cause of death that year, with 32,439 reported suicides. One suicide is committed every 17 minutes in the United States. Suicide accounts for $25 billion in direct costs in the United States. Firearms are involved in 51.6% of completed suicides in the United States. Suicide occurs in all socioeconomic groups, and it is preventable.[1]

Eighty percent of patients who commit suicide have a mood disorder, and 25% are alcohol-dependent. Suicide is the cause of death for 15% of people in those two groups. Ten percent of patients with schizophrenia die by suicide. Although patients with psychiatric disorders have a higher rate of suicide, an underlying disorder does not have to be present.

The common acronym "SAD PERSONS" aids in identifying patients at increased risk for suicide (Table 6.1).

Other risk factors for suicide include race, religious preference, family history of suicide, and past physical or sexual abuse. Non-Hispanic whites and American Indians have the highest rates of suicide, while non-Hispanic blacks, Asian and Pacific Islanders, and Hispanics have the lowest rates. In terms of religion, Protestants and Jews have higher rates of suicide than Catholics and Muslims. Patients with a family history of suicide or who have been directly exposed to suicide or suicide attempts have an increased risk of suicide. People exposed to media coverage of suicide attempts are at higher risk for suicide.

All forms of substance abuse and dependence increase the risk of suicide. Actual intoxication at the time of the suicide is common. The risk for alcoholic persons is particularly high in the 6 months after a major loss.

Table 6.1 "SAD PERSONS"	
S	Sex (attempts female:male = 3:1, completion female:male = 1:>3)*
A	Age (bimodal, with adolescents and elderly persons at greatest risk)
D	Depression or other psychiatric disorder
P	Previous suicide attempts
E	Alcohol (Ethanol) or drug use
R	Rational thinking loss (e.g., in psychosis)
O	Organized plan
S	Social supports lacking
N	No spouse (divorced, widowed, separated, single), no children
S	Sickness (chronic, debilitating, severe)

* Females are more likely to attempt suicide, but males are more likely to die from their suicidal attempt.

Source: Patterson WM, Dohn HH, Bird J, Patterson GA. Evaluation of suicidal patients: the SAD PERSONS scale. *Psychosomatics*. 1983;24(4):343–345, 348–349.

Suicide attempts are greater in females, while completed suicide rates are higher in males. Any past history of suicidal behavior dramatically increases the risk for a future completed suicide.

The patient most likely to commit suicide is an elderly white man with no social supports, so special vigilance is needed in this patient population.[2]

Suicide evaluation and management

There is no reason not to assess patients for SI. Asking about suicide does not "plant" the idea in a patient's mind, nor does it increase its probability. Any patient with SI needs an immediate referral to the mental health system (refer to Chapter 2, "When to Call for Psychiatric Help").

SI needs to be evaluated in terms of frequency, intent, and plan. Although many people occasionally experience a stray suicidal thought, constant, frequent, or powerful suicidal thoughts are not normal. If a patient does experience current or recurrent thoughts of suicide, he or she should be asked about any plans for suicide. Finally, if the patient is actively thinking of suicide and has made a plan, it is important to determine the patient's intent to carry out the plan. During the evaluation, ensure the patient's safety: do not leave the patient alone, and remove any potentially dangerous objects from the room.

For a patient who has just made a suicide attempt, assess whether the attempt was planned or impulsive; determine the lethality of the attempt, the chance that the patient's action might be discovered, the reaction to the patient's survival, and whether the factors that led to the attempt have changed.

Emergency psychiatric evaluation may be required, possibly including involuntary commitment proceedings.

The clinician must be aware of personal feelings toward patients with suicidal thoughts (countertransference), especially when encountering patients with parasuicidal behaviors. It is important not to trivialize any stated suicidal ideation and to remember that further evaluation is typically required. The vigilance of health care providers, early detection, and proper treatment of contributory psychiatric disorders can be a powerful tool in decreasing rates of death by suicide.

Useful resources

World Health Report: Clarifying History. Geneva: World Health Organization; 2004.

Centers for Disease Control and Prevention. WISQARS, National Vital Statistics System. http://www.cdc.gov/ncipc/wisqars/

Centers for Disease Control and Prevention. *Suicide: Facts at a Glance*. http://www.cdc.gov/ncipc/dvp/Suicide/SuicideDataSheet.pdf

U.S. Department of Health and Human Services. National Suicide Prevention Lifeline. 800–273-TALK. http://www.suicidepreventionlifeline.org/

References

1. U.S. Department of Health and Human Services. *The Surgeon General's Call to Action to Prevent Suicide.* Available at: http://www.surgeongeneral.gov/library/calltoaction/index.html. Updated January 4, 2007. Accessed June 30, 2008.

2. Centers for Disease Control and Prevention. *Suicide Prevention.* Available at: http://www.cdc.gov/ncipc/dvp/Suicide/. Updated December 6, 2007. Accessed June 30, 2008.

3. Patterson WM, Dohn HH, Bird J, Patterson GA. Evaluation of suicidal patients: the SAD PERSONS scale. *Psychosomatics.* 1983;24(4):343–345, 348–349.

Chapter 7

The patient with depressive symptoms

Y. Pritham Raj

A quick depression screening

Detecting depression is important in the practice of medicine. Roughly one-third of the patients who walk into a clinic or hospital will have issues with depression at some point. Is there an efficient way to quickly screen for depression, even when one is three patients behind in clinic or under the gun to tuck in three new admissions on the floor?

The answer is yes. There are many ways to screen for depression, but the key is for the clinician to pick one he or she is comfortable with and then actually *use* it, even if it means simply asking the patient if he or she feels depressed. The U.S. Preventive Services Task Force (USPSTF) currently recommends formal screening for depression as a category B intervention: physicians should routinely provide the service to eligible patients; there is at least fair evidence that the intervention improves important health outcomes and that the benefits outweigh the harms.

The two-question version of the PRIME-MD Patient Health Questionnaire[1] is among the most efficient screening tools, boasting a sensitivity rate of 96% in detecting major depression compared to more elaborate screens. It is administered by asking the following two questions:

1. During the past month, have you been bothered by feeling down, depressed, or hopeless?
2. During the past month, have you often been bothered by little interest or pleasure in doing things?

Making the diagnosis

If either question is answered affirmatively, a more thorough assessment is warranted. This raises another important question: once the patient has screened positive for possible depression, is there an easy way to more thoroughly assess for depression and make a proper diagnosis?

The short answer is yes—depending on the clinician's perspective. There are shortcuts (such as using "gut instinct"), and then there are the nine official criteria for depression that, if present for a 2-week period, help make the formal diagnosis. It is advisable to use the latter method. When five of the nine criteria are met, the diagnosis is major depression. Minor depression, a diagnosis that is currently being refined for better clinical utility, can be loosely diagnosed when fewer than five of the nine criteria are met and there is some level of impairment. A helpful mnemonic for remembering the nine criteria for the diagnosis of major depressive disorder is SIGECAPS (Table 7.1).[2]

A major difficulty with these criteria, as with most in psychiatry, is that they rely largely on subjective symptoms rather than objective data. There are no meaningful lab tests, vital signs, or radiographic findings to guide the assessment or treatment of depression. Additionally, patients often find it difficult to provide "yes" or "no" answers when queried about specific depressive symptoms. This is where spectrum rating scales such as the full Primary Care Evaluation of Mental Disorders Patient Health Questionnaire-9 (PRIME-MD PHQ-9; Fig. 7.1) can be of great value.

The PHQ-9 does not only help screen for depression; it can also help make a formal diagnosis. Its validity has been assessed against an independent structured mental health professional interview. A PHQ-9 score of at least 10 has been found to have a sensitivity of 88% and a specificity of 88% for major depression.[3] Of equal importance, the score can also be used to measure treatment response over time. It can be helpful to automate the administration of the PHQ-9, such as by having an assistant ask each patient to complete the scale before the physician even enters the room.

Whenever a patient reports suicidal ideation or thoughts of death, this should trigger a thorough and systematic safety evaluation as discussed in the psychiatric emergencies section of this text (refer to Chapter 5, "Psychiatric Emergencies").

Differential diagnosis of depressive symptoms

The following list is intended not to be complete but rather to highlight the common competing diagnoses and reasons why each must be

Table 7.1 SIGECAPS mnemonic for depression

* **D**epressed mood—most of the day and nearly every day by subjective or objective account
* **S**leep (insomnia or hypersomnia)
* **I**nterests that are markedly diminished (anhedonia)
* **G**uilt (includes sense of worthlessness)
* **E**nergy loss/fatigue
* **C**oncentration (poor)
* **A**ppetite (5% loss or gain from baseline in a month)
* **P**sychomotor agitation or retardation
* **S**uicidal ideation/thoughts of death

PATIENT HEALTH QUESTIONAIRE (PHQ-9)

NAME: _____ DATE: _____

Over the *last 2 weeks*, how often have you been
bothered by any of the following problems?
(use " ✓" to indicate your answer)

	Not at all	Several days	More than half the days	Nearly every day
1. Little interest or pleasure in doing things	0	1	2	3
2. Feeling down, depressed, or hopeless	0	1	2	3
3. Trouble falling or staying asleep, or sleeping too much	0	1	2	3
4. Feeling tired or having little energy	0	1	2	3
5. Poor appetite or overeating	0	1	2	3
6. Feeling bad about yourself—or that you are a failure or have let yourself or your family down	0	1	2	3
7. Trouble concentrating on things, such as reading the newspaper or watching television	0	1	2	3
8. Moving or speaking so slowly that other people could have noticed. Or the opposite—being so fidgety or restless that you have been moving around a lot more than usual	0	1	2	3
9. Thoughts that you would be better off dead, or of hurting yourself in some way	0	1	2	3

add columns: ___ + ___ + ___

(Healthcare professional: For interpretation of TOTAL, please refer to accompanying scoring card). TOTAL: ___

10. If you checked off *any* problems, how *difficult* have these problems made it for you to do your work, take care of things at home, or get along with other people?

Not difficult at all _____
Somewhat difficult _____
Very difficult _____
Extremely difficult _____

Figure 7.1 Patient Health Questionnaire (PHQ-9). Developed by Drs. Robert L. Spitzer, Janet B. Williams, and Kurt Kroenke. Copyright © Pfizer Inc. All rights reserved.

considered when assessing the depressed patient. Most of them are covered in other sections of this text (refer to Chapter 8, "The Patient with Manic Symptoms," Chapter 10, "The Patient with Disordered Use of Substances or Alcohol," Chapter 13, "The Patient with Confusion or Memory Problems," and Chapter 17, "The Geriatric Patient").

1. **Bipolar Disorder**—This is perhaps the most important psychiatric disorder to consider when evaluating the depressed patient. A bipolar patient may look very depressed. In fact, 60% of people with bipolar disorder are in the depressed phase when they go to their primary care physician for help. Moreover, up to 30% of primary care patients treated for depression and/or anxiety actually have bipolar disorder. This is problematic, because if antidepressants are prescribed to patients with bipolar disorder instead of the more appropriate mood stabilizers,

there is a 30% chance of precipitating manic symptoms as a result. The screening for bipolar disorder is therefore essential when evaluating the depressed patient. The Bipolar Spectrum Diagnostic Scale (BSDS)[4] is a helpful tool for screening for mania. It takes the form of a narrative paragraph that is easy to read—and one that bipolar patients typically identify with rather strongly. Again, it is less important *how* one screens than *that* one does screen systematically for bipolar disorder.

2. **Substance Abuse/Dependence**—The effects of many illicit and pre-scription drugs, as well as withdrawal states, mimic depression. It is important to assess and treat these conditions before adding pharma-cotherapy for depression, which could make the patient worse. One of the most underappreciated causes of serotonin syndrome occurs when certain opiates are used in conjunction with serotonin reuptake inhibitors.

3. **Bereavement**—Both grief (the subjective feeling following a death or loss) and bereavement (the state of being deprived by a death or loss) are normal reactions. However, when symptoms persist for longer than 2 months, the diagnosis of depression must be enter-tained. This can be viewed similarly to the way in which a patient with an adjustment reaction to a given stressor either goes on to resolu-tion or toward a full depressive episode over time.

4. **Medical/Physical Disorders**—There is an exhaustive list of medical disorders that can be associated with depression, including a variety of malignancies, infectious diseases (especially HIV), rheumatologic disorders, cardiac disease, and more recently even vitamin deficien-cies such as of vitamin D.[5] However, the endocrinopathies have some of the most intimate association with depressive illness. Diabetes is a major one, but two others that are less heralded but important not to overlook are the following:

    i. **Thyroid Disease**—Checking a thyroid-stimulating hormone (TSH) level is common when evaluating for cognitive disorders and anx-iety spectrum illness. Yet depression can also be associated with thyroid disease, often rendering TSH screening useful. When depressive symptoms accompany subclinical thyroid dysfunction, optimal management is not entirely clear. Observation may be the best strategy because although perhaps easy to treat, one study noted no real association between subclinical thyroid disease and depression—or anxiety or cognition for that matter. Typically, it is reasonable not to treat subclinical hypothyroidism (the key con-cern in depression) until the TSH rises above 10 mIU/L or there are other compelling reasons to do so.[6]

    ii. **Hypogonadism**—The subject of much controversy, dehydroepi-androsterone (DHEA) deficiency and testosterone deficiency are often overlooked in the workup of depressive symptoms despite the frequent association with low mood. Aging and a variety of other medical illnesses have been implicated in androgen defi-ciency, with newer studies showing the efficacy of replacement when treating associated mood symptoms.[7]

5. **Cognitive Disorders**—*Pseudodementia* refers to cognitive changes that are thought to be the direct result of depression (or other mood disorders). Conversely, cognitive disorders such as dementia and delirium can certainly mimic depression. In an analysis of psychiatric consultations performed at Duke University Medical Center, about one-eighth of patients with delirium were mistakenly called in as consults for the treatment of depression.

6. **Anxiety Spectrum Illness**—Depression and anxiety are intimately connected. If one examines the somatic symptoms of generalized anxiety disorder (GAD) in the *DSM-IV-TR*,[8] as outlined in Table 7.2 in the TICKES mnemonic that I created as a memory tool to help remember the GAD criteria, it is plain to see how much symptom overlap there is with depression. Although the treatments for depression and anxiety tend to be the same (primarily the second-generation antidepressants), controlling anxiety symptoms tends to require higher dosing than treating depression alone (refer to Chapter 4, "Overview of Psychopharmacologic Therapies").

7. **Personality Disorders**—Affective instability, a cardinal feature of depression, is also a key feature of borderline personality disorder (BPD). A recent evidence-based review discusses the key features and treatment options for BPD[9] (also refer to Chapter 21, "Overview of the Practice of Psychotherapy").

Treatment strategies

Clinical scenario 1

After careful assessment, a patient appears to have unipolar major depression. She agrees with the diagnosis but wants to know the best way to treat her symptoms. What is the best next step—is medication the obvious next choice?

Not necessarily. Even though 60% to 80% of patients will respond to pharmacotherapy (that tends to work fastest), other treatments can be effective and have been well accepted. The speed-of-efficacy data are important because the longer a treatment for depression takes, the lower

Table 7.2 **TICKES mnemonic for generalized anxiety disorder**
Generalized Anxiety Disorder (GAD): in addition to difficulty controlling worry, at least 3 of the following are required over a 6-month period:
• **T**ension in muscles
• **I**rritability
• **C**oncentration is poor
• **K**eyed up/restless
• **E**asily fatigued
• **S**leep disturbance

the chances for remission. Additionally, the longer the episode of depression, the greater the brain atrophy—a set-up for future cognitive impairment and so forth. Still, an important treatment of depression centers on lifestyle modification, specifically an exercise regimen.

Exercise

Jumping to pharmacotherapy before discussing exercise is like giving a patient with type 2 diabetes mellitus night-time insulin before providing nutrition counseling. Such a plan would be flawed. If a depressed patient simply sits on his couch watching television all day, the use of an antidepressant will have a far smaller chance of working than if the patient were physically active. In fact, according to the original SMILE (Standard Medical Intervention and Long-term Exercise) study comparing medications to exercise (using a stationary bicycle, walking, or jogging for 30 minutes three times per week), although sertraline was a little faster in leading to remission, the remission rate of 65.5% with medication was statistically no different than the 60.4% rate for patients in the exercise group.[10] Longer-term continuation studies confirmed lasting benefits to exercise. Hence, exercise is an effective primary treatment for depression.

Pharmacotherapy

Medication options are covered in Chapter 4, "Overview of Psychopharmacologic Therapies," and there are excellent reviews on the subject elsewhere.[11] But it is important to briefly review the largest antidepressant trial to date, the Sequenced Treatment Alternatives to Relieve Depression (STAR*D) study sponsored by the National Institute of Mental Health.[12,13] Choosing a medication to treat depression is often a conundrum, with big pharmaceutical companies flooding the media with reasons why their drug is the best choice.

Medications such as venlafaxine and mirtazapine have demonstrated promise when it comes to speed of efficacy. However, when considering basic rates of remission, the primary goal in the treatment of depression, the first two levels of the STAR*D trial showed that even if a patient's depression did not remit with initial SSRI treatment (in this case citalopram, which had a nearly 30% remission rate), there was no real difference in remission rates when a monotherapy switch was made, regardless of class of antidepressant used—with venlafaxine XR, bupropion SR, and sertraline showing similar efficacy.[12] The second phase[13] highlighted the similar rates of efficacy of augmentation (with either bupropion SR, buspirone, or cognitive therapy) when monotherapy with an SSRI failed to lead to remission. Practically speaking, if patients do not show at least 30% improvement in symptoms on a medication, consider switching. If a medication leads to 30% improvement or more but depressive symptoms are still problematic, consider augmentation (refer to Chapter 4, "Overview of Psychopharmacologic Therapies").

For patients who prefer alternative pharmacotherapy, two of the better-studied herbs and supplements include St. John's wort (*Hypericum perforatum*) and chromium picolinate, respectively. St. John's wort has been shown to have benefit in mild to moderate depression, while chromium has been shown to have both mood and metabolic benefits in small studies to date.[14]

How long should pharmacotherapy be continued once a depressive episode is under control? There are no clear data to answer this. Most consensus guidelines recommend at least a year of treatment before discontinuation is attempted. The minimum length of treatment for a first episode of major depression should be at least 6 months. For patients who have had two episodes of depression previously, the recommendation is to continue treatment indefinitely.

Referral to psychiatry

As a general rule, given the drop-off in efficacy in the latter stages of the STAR*D trial, if a patient fails to respond to more than two or three antidepressant trials, it is prudent to refer him or her for specialty care. Many non-psychiatrists feel uncomfortable prescribing medications such as lithium and antipsychotics, which, among others, are considered as augmentation strategies in the treatment of depression.

Psychotherapy or "talk" therapy

There is controversy about the merits of psychotherapy compared to pharmacotherapy, but there is little debate about the benefit of the two treatments used in combination. Hence, psychotherapy should be recommended to all patients who are depressed and have stressors that would benefit from supportive therapy or maladaptive behaviors for which cognitive restructuring would help (refer to Chapter 21, "Overview of the Practice of Psychotherapy"). The only drawback is that psychotherapy typically takes longer than pharmacotherapy to alleviate symptoms. In reality, lack of insurance benefit and/or cost tends to be the limiting factor when considering psychotherapy as a treatment option.

Electroconvulsive therapy (ECT) or "electric shock" therapy

This emotionally (and electrically) charged treatment has been the subject of great debate since its introduction in the 1930s, yet nothing has been proven more effective in the treatment of depression. The nature of the therapy—passing electrical current through the scalp to generate a convulsive seizure—is often cited as the reason for refusal by patients who do not elect ECT, despite the fact that it is performed in a controlled environment under general anesthesia. Science is still unable to fully explain how ECT works, but according to historical data it boasts an unmatched 90% efficacy rate in the treatment of depression. Regarding its mechanism of action, it can be helpful to describe ECT to patients in computer terms—likening it to a "reboot" of the malfunctioning brain. Also used in the treatment of bipolar disorder, schizophrenia, and some neurological disorders, its most common use is in the treatment of refractory depression. Referral to a center that performs ECT is prudent for the patient who has failed to respond to conventional treatment.

Common pitfalls

1. **Diagnosis**—As mentioned in the "Differential Diagnosis" section of this chapter, the most common pitfall in making a depression diagnosis is overlooking a bipolar-spectrum illness.

2. **Treatment**—There are three major safety pitfalls with pharmacotherapy that target serotonergic pathways: suicidality, serotonin syndrome, and, to a lesser degree, abnormal bleeding.

   i. **Suicide**—In 2004, the most highly publicized concern, suicidality—defined as new or increased suicidal thoughts, preparations for attempts, or attempts—was listed by the U.S. Food and Drug Administration (FDA) under a black-box warning for patients under the age of 18. Although the warning has been recommended for extension to include patients up to age 24, it is important to remember that there have been no completed suicides linked directly to antidepressant therapy in the United States. In fact, most experts agree with the newer data that the benefits of antidepressant therapy in children and adolescents outweigh the risks. Fewer than 1 in 100 had suicidal thoughts or behaviors when taking the medications. But the biggest pitfall is not following a patient closely after medications are prescribed.

   ii. **Serotonin Syndrome**—In this syndrome there is excessive stimulation of central and peripheral serotonergic receptors, typically the result of medication excess or drug interactions, such as interactions between amitriptyline–paroxetine and tramadol–fluoxetine. Use of linezolid, furazolidone, isoniazid, and procarbazine for patients who are taking SSRIs may result in serotonin syndrome because of their nonselective MAO-inhibiting properties. Meperidine, which blocks the neuronal reuptake of serotonin, is not recommended for patients taking SSRIs. Symptoms of the syndrome can include the following:
      - Diarrhea
      - Diaphoresis
      - Tachycardia
      - Blood pressure elevation
      - Altered mental status (delirium)
      - Myoclonus
      - Increased motor activity
      - Irritability
      - Severe symptoms: hyperpyrexia, shock, death

   iii. **Abnormal Bleeding**—Since platelets use serotonin for their functioning, there is emerging concern that antidepressants with a high degree of serotonin reuptake inhibition (like fluoxetine, paroxetine, and sertraline) also have higher association with abnormal bleeding, such as gastrointestinal and dysfunctional uterine bleeding.[15] Newer data suggest that the bleeding risk is more highly correlated to concomitant NSAID use.

Useful resources

1. Depression Screening. Available at: www.ahrq.gov/research/mentalix .htm#Depression
2. The PHQ-9 Questionnaire. Available at: www.depression-primarycare .org/clinicians/toolkits/materials/forms/phq9/questionnaire/
3. Bipolar Screening. Available at: www.psycheducation.org/depression/BSDS

References

1. Whooley MA, Avins AL, Miranda J, Browner WS. Case-finding instruments for depression: two questions are as good as many. *J Gen Intern Med.* 1997; 12:439–445.
2. Carlat DJ. The psychiatric review of symptoms: a screening tool for family physicians. *Am Fam Physician.* 1998;58(7):1617–1624.
3. Spitzer RL, Kroenke K, Williams JB. Validation and utility of a self-report version of PRIME-MD: the PHQ primary care study. Primary Care Evaluation of Mental Disorders. Patient Health Questionnaire. *JAMA.* 1999;282(18):1737–1744.
4. Nassir Ghaemi S, Miller CJ, Berv DA, Klugman J, Rosenquist KJ, Pies RW. Sensitivity and specificity of a new bipolar spectrum diagnostic scale. *J Affect Disord.* 2005;84(2–3):273–277.
5. Hoogendijk WJG, Lips P, Dik MG, et al. Depression is associated with decreased 25-hydroxyvitamin D and increased parathyroid hormone levels in older adults. *Arch Gen Psychiatry.* 2008;65:508–512.
6. Roberts LM, Pattison H, Roalfe A, et al. Is subclinical thyroid dysfunction in the elderly associated with depression or cognitive dysfunction? *Ann Intern Med.* 2006;145:573–581.
7. Morsink LF, Vogelzangs N, Nicklas BJ, et al. Associations between sex steroid hormone levels and depressive symptoms in elderly men and women: results from the Health ABC study. *Psychoneuroendocrinology.* 2007; July 23 [Epub ahead of print].
8. American Psychiatric Association. *Diagnostic and Statistical Manual of Mental Disorders, 4th ed., Text Revision.* Washington, DC: American Psychiatric Association; 2000.
9. Raj YP. Psychopharmacology of borderline personality disorder. *Curr Psychiatry Rep.* 2004;6:225–231.
10. Blumenthal JA, Babyak MA, Moore KA, et al. Effects of exercise training on older patients with major depression. *Arch Intern Med.* 1999;159:2459–2456.
11. Mann JJ. The medical management of depression. *N Engl J Med.* 2005; 353:1819–1834.
12. Rush AJ, Trivedi MH, Wisniewski SR, et al. Bupropion-SR, sertraline, or venlafaxine-XR after failure of SSRIs for depression. *N Engl J Med.* 2006;354:1231–1242.
13. Trivedi MH, Fava M, Wisniewski SR, et al. Medication augmentation after the failure of SSRIs for depression. *N Engl J Med.* 2006;354:1243–1252.
14. Docherty JP, Sack DA, Roffman M, et al. A double-blind, placebo-controlled, exploratory trial of chromium picolinate in atypical depression: effect on carbohydrate craving. *J Psychiatric Practice.* 2005;11(5):302–314.
15. Meijer WEE, Heerdink ER, Nolen WA, et al. Association of risk of abnormal bleeding with degree of serotonin reuptake inhibition by antidepressants. *Arch Intern Med.* 2004;164:2367–2370.

Chapter 8

The patient with manic symptoms

Yeshesvini Raman

Clinical scenario

BT is a 24-year-old woman who recently moved from California to study at Duke University. Her friends have always known her to be a high-spirited, energetic, and enthusiastic individual. She comes to the physician's office for help with sleep, as she has had very little or no sleep for the past week or so. Her final exams are just 3 weeks away, and she has been unable to focus on her studies despite feeling energetic and sharp. She does keep herself very busy during the day but cannot tell the physician what she has been doing constructively. She says, "I will definitely pass at the top of my class." When asked how she has been eating, she says, "God has asked me to eat only one fruit a day and drink four glasses of water. That is the only way I can pass my exams." Her boyfriend reports that she has been argumentative and has demonstrated "risky behaviors" such as going on a walk alone at 2 AM. Her past medical history includes a diagnosis of bipolar disorder (which she did not agree with), and she has not been taking her medications, as they interfere with her "creativity." She has a strong family history for bipolar disorder. On exam she is restless and pacing and has rapid speech that is difficult to interrupt. It is difficult to keep up with the conversation.

What is "manic?"

The term "manic" is derived from *manikos*, which is Greek for mad. "Manic" is often very loosely used in practice to describe individuals who are hyperactive in speech and activity, have inappropriate behavior with elated moods, are sexually indiscriminate, and have poor ability to maintain boundaries. In addition, individuals who are in a state of agitation or frenzy can be perceived as "manic." These symptoms may be part of a bipolar spectrum of disorders and can be diagnosed as being manic only if they are not related to an underlying medical illness and if they meet *DSM-IV-TR* criteria for this particular disorder: at least a 1-week period of behaviors that create impairment in relationships or ability to work, including elevated, expansive, or irritable mood along with other symptoms such as grandiosity, pressured speech, decreased need for sleep, racing thoughts, distractibility, and engagement in activities that are either more productive or more impulsive (excessive work, sex, spending, or engaging in unadvisable business ventures).[1]

Symptoms that indicate a patient is manic

1. Feeling like "my mood is great, nothing can slow me down"
2. Mood always fluctuating—it changes from being down to being irritable and too happy
3. Grandiose thoughts of being able to do anything and everything, feeling "on top of the world" or "invincible"
4. Hyperreligious or hypersexual thoughts (engaging in chanting, praying, singing; increased sexual activity); also thoughts of being "special," having special powers to talk with God or having "healing powers"
5. Easily distractible: jumping from one activity to another and poor completion of tasks
6. Poor ability to concentrate on work/studies; concentration and attention span are poor
7. Inability to sleep or decreased need for sleep; feeling "hyper" like the "Energizer bunny"; not feeling tired despite poor sleep
8. Friends and family have difficulty keeping up with the patient's rapid speech and rapidly changing topics, thoughts, and ideas
9. Increasing risky behaviors—using alcohol or drugs, not using protection during sexual activity or involvement in high-risk sexual behavior
10. Spending too much money on things the patient does not need or cannot afford

A number of these symptoms may be brought to the patient's and physician's attention by friends and family because the patient may have very poor insight into them. Some patients also have paranoia and have significant delusions that interfere with their normal day-to-day functioning. They may also have auditory and visual hallucinations (refer to Chapter 12, "The Patient with Psychotic Symptoms").

Key elements in the mental status exam

Appearance: flamboyant clothes, heavy make-up, brightly colored clothing
Activity: increased; pacing, fidgety, stereotyped movements
Speech: rapid, pressured, difficult to interrupt
Mood: good, "on top of the world," super, irritable
Affect: elated, expansive, silly, irritable
Thought content: suicidal/homicidal ideation may be present; this needs to be screened for

Thought process: circumstantial (goes around like in a circle and comes back to the same topic); tangential (runs off on a tangent, never to come back to the topic of discussion); flight of ideas (abrupt and unrelated comments); disorganized

Perception: auditory or visual hallucinations and delusions

Insight and *Judgment*: altered, poor—the patient may have no idea that thoughts are illogical and may in fact believe that the problem lies with others

Patients presenting with manic symptoms may not have bipolar disorder

Manic symptoms are not necessarily diagnostic of bipolar disorder, manic type. Consequently, the patient may require a thorough evaluation to distinguish this from other causes that may mimic mania. A thorough screening for medical etiologies, as well as understanding and awareness of other diagnoses that have similar presentations, will assist in providing adequate treatment, preventing complications and hospitalization, and reducing morbidity. Any time a patient presents with symptoms consistent with mania, a comprehensive physical exam to rule out other diagnoses, or "secondary mania," is warranted.

Differential diagnosis for patients presenting with manic symptoms

1. **Delirium**: due to multiple factors. A quick screen by asking questions about orientation and level of consciousness can help identify this. A delirious patient will be disoriented or will have fluctuating consciousness, and in this case an underlying acute medical or toxicological cause should be sought.
2. **Medical Diagnoses**: hyperthyroidism, CNS lymphoma, CNS lupus, Parkinson's disease, CNS herpes, neurosyphilis, frontal lobe syndrome with hypersexual behavior, toxoplasmosis, HIV, Huntington's disease, hyperparathyroidism, stroke, head injury.
3. **Psychiatric Diagnoses**: Schizoaffective disorder, histrionic personality disorder, narcissistic personality disorder, post-traumatic stress disorder, borderline personality disorder, brief reactive psychosis, traumatic brain injury (TBI).
4. **Drug Intoxication**: Cocaine, PCP, amphetamines, other psychostimulants.
5. **Medications**: Steroids—the higher the dose, the more the risk; prior history of psychosis/mania can predict future risk. Other medications include antiretroviral therapy; NNRTI; ganciclovir; antidepressants in high doses—use special caution and screen before initiating antidepressants in a patient who has depressive symptoms (refer

to Chapter 4, "Overview of Psychopharmacologic Therapies," and Chapter 7, "The Patients with Depressive Symptoms").

6. **Deficiency States**: vitamin B$_{12}$.
7. **Seizure Disorders**: temporal lobe epilepsy.

It is also important to screen for comorbidities, including anxiety disorders, substance abuse or dependence, and post-traumatic stress disorder.

Though it is important to screen all patients under consideration for antidepressant therapy for history of mania, there are some clues that may lead to increased suspicion for the existence of bipolar disorder. These include the following:

1. Hospitalization for "nervous breakdown"
2. Family history of bipolar disorder
3. Nonresponse to treatment for "depression" despite adequate trials of multiple medications
4. Significant comorbid substance abuse
5. "Mood swings" or fluctuating pattern of mood
6. Multiple hospitalizations

Laboratory evaluation

The following laboratory studies should be considered:

- Complete blood counts
- Comprehensive metabolic profiles
- Thyroid screen
- Urine drug screen and blood toxicology screen
- Blood cultures × 2 (if febrile)
- Erythrocyte sedimentation rate
- CT scan/MRI

Also consider EEG and lumbar puncture with any new-onset psychosis and mania.

Treatment recommendations

In general, patients presenting with manic symptoms require emergent or urgent care—that is, an immediate workup to decide whether the patient needs to be hospitalized or may be discharged following the visit.

Hospitalization is warranted when a patient is psychotic or suicidal/homicidal, cannot function, has not been eating or sleeping, has poor insight, and/or demonstrates behavior for which the risk level is high. If the patient is unwilling to seek inpatient treatment and dangerous symptoms exist, an involuntary commitment may be required. When a medical cause is highly suspected for the presentation of "mania," admitting the patient to a medical service (ideally, a medicine and psychiatry combined service) is optimal.

In patients with mania and no other underlying cause after a thorough medical evaluation, the level of treatment depends on the degree of impairment in functioning. It is important to assess for risk for self-harm, and poor reality testing and poor insight may impede judgment (refer to Chapter 2, "When to Call for Psychiatric Help").

Mood stabilizers are the treatment of choice for long-term stabilization of mood. Some mood stabilizers are lithium, valproate, carbamazepine, and lamotrigine. Antipsychotics have also been approved for use on a long-term basis. In the initial phase they also help through their sedating action. More evidence has emerged supporting the use of typical or atypical antipsychotic medication in bipolar disorder, both for mania and for depression. Benzodiazepines also have sedative action and are helpful in controlling full-blown manic symptoms. Antidepressants can worsen the illness and their benefit has not been clearly shown, so they should be used with caution (refer to Chapter 4, "Overview of Psychopharmacologic Therapies").

In most cases, due to the complexity of illness, patients will benefit from referral to a psychiatric provider for management of the manic symptoms and their bipolar disorder.

Other treatments

In some cases, patients with persistent psychotic symptoms may require stabilization with ECT. Psychotherapy techniques, including supportive psychotherapy, psychoeducation, and cognitive-behavioral therapy, have been shown to be of benefit in aiding long-term remission of symptoms (refer to Chapter 21, "Overview of the Practice of Psychotherapy").

Reference

1. American Psychiatric Association. *Diagnostic and Statistical Manual of Mental Disorders, Fourth Edition, Text Revision* (DSM-IV-TR). Washington, DC: American Psychiatric Association; 2000.

Chapter 9

The patient with symptoms of anxiety

Eric J. Christopher

Clinical scenario

Ms. J is a 27-year-old woman who presents to the emergency room with chest pain and shortness of breath. The ED staff triages her to the chest pain protocol to rule out myocardial infarction. Vital signs reveal a blood pressure of 135/85, a heart rate of 110, respiratory rate of 18, and a normal temperature. After basic labs are collected and an ECG is obtained, Dr. C obtains further history. Ms. J reports that she was at work, preparing to make a presentation to the senior partner on her auditing team. She noticed that several key data points were missing, and she was struggling to gather the right data for the next day's meeting. While sitting at her computer, she gradually began to notice a "heaviness" in her chest and developed slight shortness of breath. These symptoms suddenly increased over the next 5 minutes to the point that she thought she was "losing it" and might die, at which point she called 911.

Background

There are 12 anxiety disorders described in the *Diagnostic and Statistical Manual of Mental Disorders, Forth Edition, Text Revision (DSM-IV-TR)*.[1] Anxiety disorders encompass a wide range of psychiatric diagnoses; can contribute to frequent emergency room visits, prolonged hospitalizations, and increased cost; and occur in as many as one-fifth of primary care patients.[2] It is therefore important for non-psychiatric physicians to screen and treat patients with anxiety disorders.

Approach to history-taking

The key feature in evaluating a patient with an anxiety disorder is conducting a thorough history and physical examination. Many medical disorders can present with symptoms similar to an anxiety disorder. Moreover, anxiety can be a harbinger of more serious disease or worsening of clinical status. Symptoms of anxiety can be very distressing to the patient and to the treatment team. To make a diagnosis of an anxiety disorder, it is important to rule out all medical conditions. Such a rule-out can seem daunting, but a well-directed interview can help to efficiently narrow the differential diagnosis.

Criteria for anxiety disorders

The *DSM-IV-TR*[1] gives diagnostic criteria for each anxiety disorder; key features of each are outlined in this section. In addition to these symptoms, the disorder must be severe enough to "cause clinically significant distress or impairment in social, occupational, or other important areas of functioning."

Acute stress disorder

- A traumatic event must be either witnessed or experienced. To qualify as traumatic, death, severe injury, or threat of integrity must occur in association with the event, and the patient must experience a sense of fear, helplessness, or horror.
- Occurs immediately and up to 30 days after the event.
- Key feature is dissociation ("shell-shocked," feeling that events are not real, lack of recall for the event).
- Additional symptom clusters include reexperiencing, hyperarousal, and avoidance.

Post-traumatic stress disorder (PTSD)

- A traumatic event has occurred as in acute stress disorder.
- Three key domains of dysfunction exist: reexperiencing, hyperarousal, and avoidance of the event or reminders of the event.
- Duration of symptoms is more than 30 days.

Generalized anxiety disorder

- Excessive anxiety and worry more days than not for at least 6 months.

Agoraphobia

- Experiences of fear that he or she will not be able to escape from a place or certain situation without embarrassment or difficulty.
- Can be accompanied by panic disorder.

Specific phobias

- Excessive or unreasonable fear of a specific situation or object (e.g., flying, dogs, heights); includes social phobia.
- Immediate anxiety response (can include a panic attack).
- Avoidance of the situation or object.

Panic attacks

- These occur during a discrete period with maximum symptom development in 10 minutes or less.
- Physiologic symptoms include palpitations, sweating, shaking, shortness of breath, choking or difficulty swallowing, chest pain, abdominal distress, paresthesias, loss of control, and thoughts of dying.

Obsessive-compulsive disorder (OCD)

- Obsessions are recurrent thoughts, images, or impulses that cause marked anxiety.
- Compulsions are actions (counting, handwashing, ordering) used to distract the patient from an obsession.
- The patient generally has good insight into the situation and realizes that the obsessions or compulsions are a product of his or her own mind.

Anxiety disorder due to a general medical condition

- A specific medical condition causes the anxiety symptoms (e.g., hyperthyroidism, pheochromocytoma); it is important to rule out such causes, as treatment for a secondary anxiety disorder requires treating the underlying cause.

Screening for anxiety disorders

Because anxiety disorders encompass a broad spectrum of psychiatric diagnoses and the time a primary care physician can spend with a patient is very limited, the following questions are recommended for a brief screening, which takes approximately 3 minutes to complete[3]:

- Are you a worrier?
- Have you ever had a panic or anxiety attack?
- Are you uncomfortable in social situations?
- Do you have any special fears, such as fear of flying, of insects, or of being on a high bridge?
- Do you have symptoms such as needing to wash your hands many times because you feel they are dirty, constantly checking things, or having annoying thoughts pop into your head repeatedly?
- Do you have dreams or memories of a terrible experience of yours, such as being attacked by someone, being in a car accident, or surviving a natural disaster?

Differential diagnosis

Panic attacks and generalized anxiety can occur in the medical setting as well as with medical illness. Most medical conditions that increase catecholamine levels can induce an inappropriate "fight or flight" response with increased physiologic responses. Specific medical disorders should be considered in the differential diagnosis and ruled out before diagnosing an anxiety disorder. Some conditions contributing to or causing anxiety include the following:

- Illicit drug use
- Metabolic abnormalities: acidosis, alkalosis, hypoglycemia
- Conditions causing hypoxia (pulmonary embolism, acute asthma/COPD)
- Endocrine disorders: hyperthyroidism, pheochromocytoma
- Cardiac conditions: myocardial infarction, arrhythmia

Treatment strategies

Treatment of anxiety varies according to the specific disorder and its severity. Both psychological and pharmacological treatments can be effective; it is important to know when each, or both, can be used. With the introduction of selective and nonselective serotonergic reuptake inhibitors (SSRIs and SNRIs), pharmacologic treatment has shifted away from the use of benzodiazepines due to their high potential for addiction and side effects.

When treating an anxiety disorder, it is important to initiate SSRIs and SNRIs at a lower dose than that used for major depression. Patients with anxiety disorders tend to be more "serotonin sensitive," and the caveat "start low and go slow" applies. In general, these medications should be started at half the starting dose for major depression (refer to Chapter 4, "Overview of Psychopharmacologic Therapies"). SNRIs are not immediately anxiolytic; they will not terminate acute anxiety. The time course for effectiveness is on the order of weeks to months. Some patients with anxiety disorders will require high doses of SSRIs. SSRIs can be effective for the treatment of agoraphobia, social phobia, panic disorder, PTSD, OCD, and GAD.

Benzodiazepines can be used to terminate an acute anxiety state or panic attack (hence their categorization as "anxiolytic" agents). They are used primarily for severe anxiety disorders. In addition, benzodiazepines can be used situationally in patients with specific phobias.

Psychological therapy is an effective treatment for many of the anxiety disorders. Different types of therapy are used depending on the condition and the patient. Some examples include cognitive-behavioral therapy (CBT), in which distorted "self" thoughts are reframed to positive experiences. Phobias and PTSD can be readily treated with exposure and desensitization therapy. Patients are gradually presented with the negative stimulus or anxiety-provoking situation through thought, imagination, or visualization, and this decreases the stress response (refer to Chapter 21, "Overview of the Practice of Psychotherapy"). Other techniques include relaxation, meditation, and other nonpharmacologic approaches (refer to Chapter 22, "Principles of Stress Management").

Anxiety in other settings

Patients may suffer from brief situational anxiety related to a number of factors. Many procedures and tests can be anxiety-inducing. Because of claustrophobia, some patients need pretreatment with a benzodiazepine before undergoing magnetic resonance imaging. In procedures such as gastroendoscopy, colonoscopy, and intubation that are uncomfortable and anxiety-provoking, conscious sedation may be needed; ultra-rapid-acting benzodiazepines can be used in a monitored setting. The patient must be monitored for oversedation, respiratory suppression, and possible idiosyncratic responses such as disinhibition with the use of benzodiazepines.

References

1. American Psychiatric Association. *Diagnostic and Statistical Manual of Mental Disorders, 4th Edition, Text Revision.* Washington, DC: American Psychiatric Association; 2000.

2. Kroenke K, Spitzer RL, Williams JB, Monahan PO, Lowe B. Anxiety disorders in primary care: prevalence, impairment, comorbidity, and detection. *Ann Intern Med.* 2007;146:317–325.

3. Carlat DJ. *The Psychiatric Interview—A Practical Guide.* Philadelphia: Lippincott Williams & Wilkins; 1999.

Chapter 10

The patient with disordered use of substances or alcohol

Glen L. Xiong

Clinical scenario

A 42-year-old woman with a history of diabetes and depression presents to establish primary care. Her key symptoms are depressed mood and insomnia. She does not keep records of her blood sugar, which is 355 at the visit. She is supposed to be taking insulin, mirtazapine, and zolpidem, but she has been out of her medication for at least 4 weeks. She lost her job 2 months ago. Divorced and living with her mother and her two teenage children, she hesitantly admits to drinking two or three glasses of wine per night and daily marijuana use. She denies any cocaine, opiate, or prescription drug abuse. She reports that she used intravenous heroin twice 10 years ago.

Background

This chapter focuses on the general approach to diagnosis and treatment of alcohol and other illicit drug (AOD) use problems as a whole, with less focus on the details of any particular substance. For simplicity, illicit drugs of abuse are divided into five major categories: cannabinoids, opiates, stimulants, hallucinogens, and inhalants.[1] Their major effects are summarized in Table 10.1.

Table 10.1 Major effects of illicit drugs	
Substance	**Mental status and physical exam**
Tetrahydrocannabinol (THC)	Impaired cognitive and motor skills; red eyes, dry mouth
Opiates	Sedation, miosis, respiratory depression
Stimulants (cocaine, amphetamine)	Elation, hyperactivity, disinhibition, delusions, hallucinations, tactile hallucinations, impulsivity, tachycardia, hypertension, diaphoresis
Hallucinogens • Serotonergic (LSD, mushrooms, mescaline)	• Vivid visual hallucinations, slurred speech, hyperarousal, ataxia, seizure

Table 10.1 *continued*	
Substance	**Mental status and physical exam**
• Anticholinergic (belladonna, jimsonweed) • Dissociative anesthetics (PCP, ketamine) • Methylated amphetamines (MDA, MDMA)	• Dreamlike trance, confusion, agitation, anticholinergic syndrome • Sense of invulnerability, nystagmus, psychosis • Aphrodisiac, "ecstasy," illusions, hallucinations
Inhalants • Volatile solvents (fingernail polish, paint thinner) • Nitrites (amyl nitrite, butyl nitrite) • General anesthetics (ether, nitrous oxide) • Aerosol gasses (hair spray, insecticides)	Disorientation, slurred speech, incoordination, illusions, lethargy

Approach to history-taking

Acutely intoxicated users usually suffer from euphoria, agitation, hallucinations, or confusion. Chronic users typically present with psychiatric symptoms such as anxiety, depression, irritability, personality disturbances, panic attacks, impaired concentration, and especially insomnia. Rarely, a patient may endorse other psychotic symptoms such as paranoia. Difficulties with managing a patient's medical conditions (as in the case scenario) should alert the physician to occult AOD use.

"At-risk" drinking is defined as more than 14 standard drinks weekly (or more than 4 drinks per occasion) for men and more than 7 drinks weekly (or 3 drinks per occasion) for women and for anyone over age 65.[2] A standard drink is defined as 1.5 oz of liquor, 12 oz of beer, or 5 oz of table wine. For other substances, there are no established guidelines about quantity.

Validated instruments that are widely accepted in clinical practice are useful for the detection of alcohol use. These include the 4-item CAGE questionnaire and the 10-item AUDIT (Alcohol Use Disorders Identification Test) questionnaire.[3] Even one affirmative answer on the CAGE (which asks whether the patient has tried to *C*ut down, has become *A*ngry when people discuss his or her drinking, whether he or she feels *G*uilty about his or her drinking, or whether he or she has ever needed an *E*ye opener) suggests need for further evaluation.[4] The AUDIT (Table 10.2) has better sensitivity and specificity than CAGE and can be completed via interview or questionnaire in as little as 2 minutes.[5] Currently, there is no standardized screening instrument for other drugs that is widely accepted.

Key points for obtaining drug and alcohol use history

Although AOD use is part of a routine comprehensive history and physical exam, patients are frequently not forthcoming about AOD habits.[6] Common reasons for denial include shame, stigma, and concern about being negatively perceived by the health care provider. It is therefore important to assure the

Table 10.2 Alcohol Use Disorders Identification Test (AUDIT)

AUDIT

Please circle the answer that is correct for you

1. How often do you have a drink containing alcohol?

| Never | Monthly or less | Two or four times a month | Two or three times a week | Four or more times a week |

2. How many drinks containing alcohol do you have on a typical day when you are drinking?

| 1 or 2 | 3 or 4 | 5 or 6 | 7 to 9 | 10 or more |

3. How often do you have six or more drinks on one occassion?

| Never | Less than monthly | Monthly | Weekly | Daily or almost daily |

4. How often during the last year have you found that you were not able to stop drinking once you had started?

| Never | Less than monthly | Monthly | Weekly | Daily or almost daily |

5. How often during the last year have you failed to do what was noramlly expected from you because of drinking?

| Never | Less than monthly | Monthly | Weekly | Daily or almost daily |

6. How often during the last year have you needed a first drink in the morning to get yourself going after a heavy drinking session?

| Never | Less than monthly | Monthly | Weekly | Daily or almost daily |

7. How often during the last year have you had a feeling of guilt or remorse after drinking?

| Never | Less than monthly | Monthly | Weekly | Daily or almost daily |

8. How often during the last year have you been unable to remember what happended the night before because you had been drinking?

| Never | Less than monthly | Monthly | Weekly | Daily or almost daily |

9. Have you or someone else been injured as a result of your drinking?

| No | | Yes, but not in the last year | | Yes, during the last year |

10. Has a relative or friend, or a doctor or other health worker been concerned about your drinking or suggested you cut down?

| No | | Yes, but not in the last year | | Yes, during the last year |

Procedure for Scoring AUDIT

Questions 1–8 are scored 0, 1, 2, 3, or 4. Questions 9 and 10 are scored 0, 2, or 4 only. The response coding is as follows:

	0	1	2	3	4
Question 1	Never	Monthly or less	Two to four times per month	Two to three times per week	Four or more times per week
Question 2	1 or 2	3 or 4	5 or 6	7 to 9	10 or more
Question 3–8	Never	Less than monthly	Monthly	Weekly	Daily or almost daily

Table 10.2 *continued*			
Question 9–10	No	Yes, but not in the last year	Yes, during the last year

The minimum score (for non-drinkers) is 0 and the maximum possible score is 40.

A score of 8 or more indicates a strong likelihood of hazadarous or harmful alcohol consumption

Reprinted with permission from Saunders JB, Aasland OG, Babor TF, de la Fuente JR, Grant M. Development of the Alcohol Use Disorders Identification Test (AUDIT): WHO Collaborative Project on Early Detection of Persons with Harmful Alcohol Consumption—II. *Addiction.* 1993;88(6):791–804. Wiley-Blackwell Publishing.

patient that the physician's role is to assist in the patient's overall health and not to judge his or her AOD problem. Noting that AOD use often adversely affects most interpersonal and family relationships and reassuring the patient about confidentiality can often decrease the patient's reluctance about bringing in close family members for support and collateral information. Patients, especially those with occult AOD use disorders and those who have not had previous treatment, may be more forthcoming after being asked if they know of family members or friends with a substance use problem and the experience with their treatment, recovery, or relapse.

Evidence of failure to fulfill family, social, or occupational roles suggests a possible AOD problem. It is important to get at least a general sense of the methods the patient may have employed to obtain drugs, particularly if they pose health risks (e.g., underground drug trade and/or prostitution). When asking about AOD use patterns, it is important to inquire about the amount of use per day, number of days of use per week, and consequent impairment in social or occupational activities.

For patients who have had treatment but have relapsed, it is important to explore any positive or negative aspects of past treatment experience. Education about the high incidence of relapse and addressing issues of shame and guilt will frequently facilitate a patient's open discussion of AOD use.

Asking open-ended questions such as "When was the last time you used…" rather than "Do you use…" will frequently result in more truthful responses, particularly when patients sense an open, nonjudgmental attitude in the health care provider.

Helpful laboratory assessment

Biomarkers for alcohol use

- Aspartate aminotransferase (AST) : alanine aminotransferase (ALT) ratio > 2
- Macrocytosis or elevated mean corpuscular volume (MCV) (specificity 85% and sensitivity 52%)
- Gamma-glutamyltransferase (GGT) (specificity 75% and sensitivity 73%)
- Carbohydrate-deficient transferrin (CDT) (specificity 92% and sensitivity 69%)[7]
- PT, PTT, and INR

Urine drug screen (UDS)

Most laboratories routinely test urine for stimulants, cocaine, opiate, benzodiazepines, and marijuana metabolites. Marijuana metabolites may be detectable days to weeks after use. Depending on the setting, some laboratories will provide a qualitative alcohol level from urine, while others require a blood sample (especially in emergency room settings). A breathalyzer is used for alcohol detection in most psychiatric and substance treatment programs. The most difficult task a provider faces is ordering a urine drug screen without appearing disrespectful. However, being too timid and underutilizing UDS in high-risk populations is irresponsible and may ultimately cause harm. A challenge for the provider is to be consistent with particular practice habits and use of objective criteria (e.g., when a particular medication is prescribed) rather than relying on subjective criteria. Each provider is prone to unique blind spots when it comes to distinguishing or "judging" those who have versus those who do not have AOD problems. Depending on the practice setting, a provider may need to develop systematic criteria for obtaining a UDS. A clinician may then tell the patient, "Generally for patients in your situation who are showing (laboratory) abnormalities for AOD use, I obtain a UDS. This is part of my practice habit because I find that most patients often have difficulty talking about AOD use." False-negatives may occur due to tampering with the collection process or when drug use occurred beyond the detectable time period. Urine specific gravity may be used to ascertain the truthfulness of the sample. False-positives occur rarely, and repeat confirmatory testing should be offered.

Differential diagnosis

It is important to rule out AOD use during the evaluation of a psychiatric disorder, violence or behavioral disturbance, suicidal ideation/attempt, and treatment resistance or nonadherence. For patients with AOD disorders, an underlying comorbid psychiatric disorder often exists, most commonly depressive, anxiety, and antisocial personality disorders.[8] The following list includes conditions that should be considered and carefully evaluated in patients with AOD disorders:

- Alcohol withdrawal seizures and delirium tremens
- Intracranial bleeding
- Sexually transmitted infections
- Blood-borne infections (HCV and HIV)
- Wernicke-Korsakoff syndrome
- Abscess and endocarditis (in injection drug users)
- Affective and anxiety disorders
- Psychotic disorders
- Suicidal and homicidal ideation

Treatment strategies

Detoxification

Pharmacological detoxification (Table 10.3) is usually employed and is often necessary for patients with physiological dependence on alcohol, benzodiazepines (BZP), and opiates. For alcohol and BZP dependence, symptom-triggered therapy using the revised Clinical Institute Withdrawal Assessment for Alcohol (CIWA-Ar) could be used for patients requiring hospitalization, although a BZP taper is more commonly employed, as most providers outside of specialized detoxification units do not have sufficient experience or training with CIWA. For a patient with a history of withdrawal seizure or underlying seizure diathesis, use of anticonvulsants such as phenytoin and valproate may be added to the BZP taper. The dose and duration of BZP taper required to prevent seizures and/or treat delirium tremens typically correlates with a patient's tolerance to alcohol and may be several times higher than the average tapering dose and treatment duration (4 days).

For opiate addiction, unless a patient is going to receive opiate maintenance therapy (methadone or buprenorphine), a clonidine taper is used for cravings and autonomic instability. Symptom-targeted medications include dicyclomine (10 to 20 mg every 6 hours as needed) for abdominal cramps, loperamide (Imodium) for diarrhea, lorazepam for restlessness, and trazodone for insomnia. For stimulant intoxication, the safety of both the patient and those caring for him or her is the number one priority. The patient may require medications and hospitalization (refer to Chapter 11, "The Patient with Agitated Symptoms," and Chapter 12, "The Patient with Psychotic Symptoms").

Table 10.3 Detoxification and maintenance of sobriety		
	Detoxification*	**Maintenance**
Alcohol and BZPs	Lorazepam (Ativan) 2 mg tid or qid	Naltrexone 50 mg daily
	Chlordiazepoxide (Librium) 25 tid or qid	Acamprosate 666 mg tid
	Symptom-triggered BZP administration	Disulfiram 250 to 500 mg daily
	Generally done in closely supervised or hospital settings	
Opiates	Clonidine 0.1 mg bid or tid	Methadone***
	Buprenorphine**	Buprenorphine**
		Buprenorphine/naloxone**

* Generally administered in a closely supervised addiction treatment program or hospital settings and tapered cautiously based on vital signs and symptoms.

** Can be prescribed after training and receiving special DEA license.

*** Can be prescribed only in licensed methadone maintenance programs.

Sobriety

Brief intervention has been shown to be effective for the treatment of problem drinking in primary care settings in four 15-minute weekly sessions. There are five key elements: (1) assessment and direct feedback (where the provider expresses concern about the patient's drinking problem), (2) negotiation and goal setting (where patient and provider agree on a mutually acceptable goal), (3) behavioral modification (where the provider helps the patient identify and avoid triggers and develop coping skills during high-risk situations), (4) self-help bibliotherapy, and (5) follow-up and reinforcement.[9] In counseling a patient to achieve abstinence, providers should assess a patient's readiness to change and choose specific targets for change. A directive yet nonconfrontational style or method called motivational interviewing using the Transtheoretical Stages of Change model (Table 10.4) has been shown to be effective in a variety of settings.[10] Different treatment approaches, including cognitive-behavioral therapy (CBT), motivational enhancement therapy (MET), and 12-step facilitation (TSF), have been found to be efficacious and equivalent for most patients.[11]

A variety of psychosocial programs, such as Alcoholics Anonymous (AA), exist to help a patient maintain abstinence. Involvement in a psychosocial program is associated with improved long-term outcomes, though in some cases a stable social environment such as established employment and a supportive family/social network may be sufficient. Family and friends might be mobilized, with the patient's consent, to facilitate access to community resources and act as chaperones. For a patient who is unemployed and has minimal psychosocial support, it is reasonable to encourage participation in a community substance abuse program either for vocational rehabilitation or as a source of primary support.

Table 10.4 Transtheoretical Stages of Change Model	
Stage	**Goals and motivational interviewing strategies**
Precontemplation	Develop a recognition that change is necessary without increasing patient resistance
	Provide education on negative consequences in a nonjudgmental way
Contemplation	Explore ambivalence by patient
	Support patient's self-motivating statements
Preparation	Provide menu of options for change
	Set "quit date" or other specific goals
Action	Praise and reinforce positive gains
	Enlist additional support resources as needed
Maintenance	Help patient acclimate to new, healthy lifestyle
	Identify potential triggers and develop relapse-prevention plan
Relapse	Explore feelings of hopelessness, guilt, or shame
	Encourage patient to reenter change cycle

Source: Hettema J, Steele J, Miller WR. Motivational interviewing. *Ann Rev Clin Psychol.* 2005;1:91–111.

Psychosocial treatments remain the fundamental treatment for substance use disorders. Most pharmacological trials are conducted with a psychosocial component. Without this, medication alone has a low probability of success. Pharmacological options for alcoholism include the opioid antagonist naltrexone (50 mg daily), the glutamate antagonist acamprosate (666 mg tid), and the acetaldehyde dehydrogenase inhibitor disulfiram (250 to 500 mg daily). For opiate dependence, traditionally a patient who is interested in long-term opiate maintenance was referred to a federally licensed methadone maintenance program. Now, a patient may be maintained on buprenorphine by a physician who undergoes training and obtains a special DEA license to prescribe buprenorphine.

Since psychiatric symptoms may resolve after abstinence is achieved, many patients and their providers decide not to start a psychotropic medication immediately following abstinence. However, psychiatric comorbidity is extraordinarily high. In practice, it is often difficult to attribute a patient's symptoms to AOD or to a primary psychiatric disorder. The provider could enlist the patient's help and discuss whether to start treating a particular psychiatric disorder when diagnostic uncertainly is high. Treatment of associated psychiatric conditions (e.g., depression) has been shown to reduce substance use.[12] In difficult cases, consultation with a psychiatrist and/or addiction medicine specialist should be considered.

Common pitfalls

Most patients who have undergone AOD programs have been educated about cross-addiction and advised to inform their physicians that particular medications (such as BZP and opiates) should be avoided. Therefore, when a patient is requesting medications with a high potential of abuse, it is important to inquire whether taking such medication is consistent with his or her goals of maintaining sobriety. It is also the medical professional's responsibility to recognize the risks and benefits of certain medications and to find alternatives whenever possible. Careless prescription of medications runs the high risk of precipitating a patient's AOD addiction—violating the Hippocratic Oath, *prima non nocere*. Remember that medications can be abused directly or bartered on the streets for the patient's drug of

Symptoms	Common pitfalls	Solution
Table 10.5 Common pitfalls in treatments involving prescription medication		
Anxiety	Benzodiazepine (BZP)	
	• May lead to dependence and misuse and facilitation of alcohol dependence	• Refer for nonpharmacological treatment of anxiety
	• Can be fatal if concurrently used with alcohol	• Use BZP taper with clear instructions and explanation of risks
	• May be used to accentuate stimulant abuse	• Consider UDS to screen for AOD problem

Symptoms	Common pitfalls	Solution
Table 10.5 *continued*		
Insomnia	• Prescription of non-BZP hypnotic • Many hypnotics have potential for physical if not psychological dependence, and there is an FDA black-box warning on driving and memory impairment	• Review and address sleep hygiene • Consider brief use of "low-risk" sleep aids such as trazodone or ramelteon (Rozerem) (refer to Chapter 15, "The Patient with Disordered Sleep")
Fatigue; attention-deficit/ hyperactivity disorder (ADHD)	• Amphetamine stimulants	• Review sleep habits and medical causes (obstructive sleep apnea) • Consider nonpharmacological treatments and pharmacological alternatives (atomoxetine, bupropion) for ADD • Obtain objective collateral information to confirm ADD • Consider UDS and use of "stimulant contract"
Pain	• Use of opiates without warning about potential for opiate dependence relapse or follow-up • Insufficient treatment of acute pain in patients on opiate maintenance	• Use non-opiate when possible • Close monitoring and follow-up and open discussion about high risk of relapse • Adequately address pain by using higher-than-average doses of short-acting opiate • Consider temporarily holding buprenorphine treatment • Use UDS and/or quantitative measure of opiate levels

choice. Table 10.5 lists specific symptoms that are likely to be encountered, as well as suggested solutions.

References

1. Johnson MD, Heriza TJ, St. Dennis C. How to spot illicit drug abuse in your patients. *Postgrad Med.* 1999;106(4):199–218.

2. National Institute on Alcohol Abuse and Alcoholism. *Helping Patients Who Drink Too Much: A Clinician's Guide* (updated edition). Bethesda, MD: Author; 2005. Available at: http://pubs.niaaa.nih.gov/publications/Practitioner/CliniciansGuide2005/guide.pdf

3. Fiellin DA, Reid MC, O'Connor PG. Screening for alcohol problems in primary care: a systematic review. *Arch Intern Med.* 2000;160:1977–1989.

4. Ewing JA. The CAGE questionnaire. *JAMA.* 1984;252:1905–1907.

5. Saunders JB, Aasland OG, Babor TF, de la Fuente JR, Grant M. Development of the Alcohol Use Disorders Identification Test (AUDIT): WHO Collaborative Project on Early Detection of Persons with Harmful Alcohol Consumption—II. *Addiction.* 1993;88(6):791–804.

6. Enoch MA, Goldman D. Problem drinking and alcoholism: diagnosis and treatment. *Am Fam Phys.* 2002;65:3:441–448.

7. Bell H, Tallaksen CM, Try K, et al. Carbohydrate-deficient transferrin and other markers of high alcohol consumption: a study of 502 patients admitted consecutively to a medical department. *Alcohol Clin Exp Res.* 1994;18:1103–1108.

8. Compton WM, Thomas YF, Stinson FS, Grant BF. Prevalence, correlates, disability, and comorbidity of DSM-IV drug abuse and dependence in the United States: results from the National Epidemiologic Survey on Alcohol and Related Conditions. *Arch Gen Psychiatry.* 2007;64(5):566–576.

9. Fleming M, Manwell LB. Brief intervention in primary care settings. A primary treatment method for at-risk, problem, and dependent drinkers. *Alcohol Res Health.* 1999;23:128–137.

10. Hettema J, Steele J, Miller WR. Motivational interviewing. *Ann Rev Clin Psychol.* 2005;1:91–111.

11. Project MATCH Research Group. Project MATCH secondary a priori hypotheses. *Addiction.* 1997;92:1671–1698.

12. Cornelius JR, Salloum IM, Ehler JG, et al. Fluoxetine in depressed alcoholics. A double-blind, placebo-controlled trial. *Arch Gen Psychiatry.* 1997;54:700–705.

Chapter 11

The patient with agitated symptoms

Wei Jiang and Jane P. Gagliardi

Clinical scenario 1

Dr. V, a physician trained in internal medicine and psychiatry, receives a request to evaluate Mr. S, a 75-year-old African American man with a history of dementia. Mr. S was sent to a skilled nursing facility (SNF) 2 weeks earlier when his wife was no longer able to take care of him. At the SNF he became agitated, uncooperative, and combative, striking a staff member. He was brought to the emergency department and admitted to General Medicine for management of agitation.

Mr. S's workup reveals bilateral lung masses and a score on the Mini-Mental State Examination (MMSE) of 5/30. His family decides not to pursue aggressive diagnostic evaluation for likely lung cancer and requests palliative care. The General Medicine team is having a hard time finding placement, as Mr. S continues to be agitated and combative despite as-needed use of antipsychotic medications and intermittent physical restraints. Dr. V's examination reveals an elderly man, sedated and restrained; his nurse tells Dr. V that Mr. S will swing his arms and kick at staff members whenever he wakes up. After a thorough discussion with the family regarding risks and rationale, Dr. V recommends a scheduled regimen of low-dose antipsychotic medications, and Mr. S's agitation improves significantly on this regimen.

Clinical scenario 2

Ms. L, a 38-year-old Asian immigrant, was reportedly eating in a restaurant at a local farmer's market when she became angry and argumentative toward the wait staff, who she believed had served people standing after her in line. The situation escalated when police arrived and she began to shout and make threatening gestures. She was handcuffed and brought to the emergency department, her fourth such visit in a year, for management of agitation. She had previously been diagnosed with psychotic disorder not otherwise specified (NOS), versus bipolar disorder. Her English is limited, and Dr. J, a physician who speaks Ms. L's native language, eventually learns that the patient suffers from chronic depression with paranoia. It appears that Ms. L's agitation is best explained by this depression and difficulty adjusting to American life. She becomes much less agitated after engaging in a course of antidepressants, atypical antipsychotics, and psychotherapy.

Background

Agitation, a state of excessive psychomotor activity accompanied by increased tension and irritability, is a cluster of nonspecific symptoms of one or more physical or psychological processes in which screaming, shouting, complaining, moaning, cursing, pacing, fidgeting, or wandering pose risk or discomfort, become disruptive or unsafe, or interfere with the delivery of care.

Agitation may be caused by a broad spectrum of conditions from severe medical or mental illness to apparently good health in a person under extreme stress. Agitation can occur suddenly or gradually. Extreme agitation can lead to confusion, hyperactivity, and outright hostility. Agitation by itself may not have much clinical significance, but if it presents with other symptoms, it can be a good indicator of a disease state. Management of agitation may therefore differ greatly, as it depends on the cause.

Causes of agitation or aggression

Agitated or aggressive behavior may be the manifestation of a wide variety of medical, neurologic, or psychiatric disorders. Numerous medical conditions, drug intoxication or withdrawal, or circumstances that worsen a person's ability to think can result in agitation. The etiology of agitation or aggression is usually found in one or more of five broad categories:

1. Dementia or cognitive impairment
2. Delirium due to a general medical condition
3. Drug intoxication or withdrawal
4. Psychotic disorder or other significant psychiatric disorder (e.g., mania)
5. Personality disorder or disruptive traits (refer to Chapter 18, "The 'Difficult' Patient")

The patient's age may serve as a guide when considering the potential etiology of agitated behavior. Delirium, dementia, and drugs (including polypharmacy or anticholinergic medications) are likely causes in the elderly, while substance abuse and personality disorders are more common in the younger population. Though rare, temporal lobe epilepsy may be a cause of psychosis and aggressive behavior.[1]

Approach to the patient with agitation

It is important to conduct a thorough diagnostic workup to exclude medical illness in any patient who presents with aggressive or agitated behavior, but assessing and ensuring the safety of the patient and staff is the first priority. Evaluation should include the following:

- Safety assessment
- Mental status examination
- Clinical history, including collateral information from family or others (coworkers, caregivers)
- Substance or drug use history
- Physical examination (including a neurologic evaluation)—vital signs may be abnormal given the sympathetic surge associated with agitation
- Review of all medications—encourage family members to bring in all medications to which the patient has access
- Laboratory studies, including complete blood count, routine chemistries, thyroid hormones, urine analysis, and drug screen of urine and blood

Other studies may be indicated based on the findings of the history and examination. A noncontrast head CT may be performed to rule out hemorrhage, stroke, or acute intracranial abnormality. Disorientation, incoherence, or a presentation involving focal neurologic symptoms suggests an underlying medical etiology or drug intoxication or withdrawal. Gross disorganization with hallucinations, delusions, or impaired thought process in an oriented patient suggests psychosis.

Agitated patients may be too intoxicated, confused, or uncooperative to immediately undergo appropriate assessments. A calm, peaceful, and nonjudgmental approach will work best; pressuring the patient into a diagnostic workup may exacerbate agitation. A quiet setting with adequate but soft lighting and one-on-one observation for redirection and safety can be very helpful. Clear, directed limit-setting will facilitate patient comfort and comprehension. When other interventions fail, physical or even chemical restraint may be necessary for patients who are combative or aggressive. These measures are not routinely recommended—they require continuous monitoring and careful documentation of vital signs and physical examination to avoid harm to the patient and should be avoided whenever possible. When patients are agitated and a personality disorder, psychosis, or substances are at play, the presence of police or security staff may be the most effective intervention.

Medications for aggressive behaviors associated with acute agitation

Not every patient presenting with agitation requires immediate treatment with medication. Figure 11.1 outlines agitation workup and management. The ultimate elimination of agitation results from successful treatment of underlying medical or psychiatric illnesses (refer to related chapters of the manual and other psychiatric textbooks for management of psychiatric etiology of agitation). Dopamine receptor antagonists (DRA) and benzodiazepines (BZP) are used for the immediate control of agitated and violent behavior.

The high-potency DRAs that cause little sedation and few anticholinergic side effects (e.g., haloperidol or fluphenazine, both equipotent) are

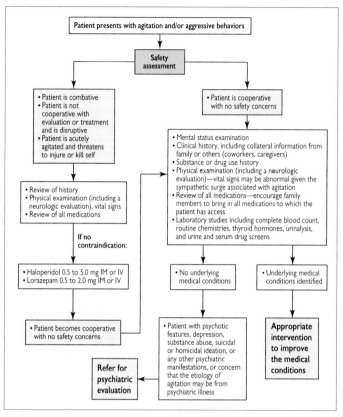

Figure 11.1 Agitation management algorithm.

preferred to the more sedating, low-potency DRAs. For mild agitation, 0.5 to 2.0 mg of haloperidol (PO or IM) is probably sufficient; higher doses can be used for more moderate or severe symptoms (2.0 to 5.0 mg). Elderly patients should be treated with lower doses (0.5 to 1.0 mg). The drug should be allowed at least 30 minutes to work before a dose is repeated. This is particularly important because akathisia, a common acute side effect of antipsychotic medications, may increase the appearance of agitation and can be exacerbated by further administration of the DRA. Although not approved for IV use, haloperidol is commonly administered IV. All antipsychotics can cause prolongation of the QTc interval and increase the risk of torsades de pointes; it is important to check and monitor ECG for QTc changes.

Low doses of lorazepam (0.5 to 2.0 mg) or diazepam (5 to 10 mg) PO, IM, or IV can produce a rapid decrease in agitation with minimal side effects. BZPs are helpful for the treatment of autonomic hyperactivity due to cocaine or other stimulants. They also may decrease anxiety in patients with acute hallucinogen or PCP intoxication, in which case all medications with anticholinergic properties must be avoided (in these cases, it is advisable to use a high-potency DRA such as haloperidol along with a BZP such as lorazepam). However, they are respiratory depressants and should be used with caution in patients who already may have a suppressed respiratory drive (e.g., in patients with chronic obstructive pulmonary disease). BZPs can also cause behavioral disinhibition.[2,3]

Often a combination of a DRA and a BZP is used to achieve more rapid results[4] and reduce acute dystonia or extrapyramidal symptoms caused by DRAs.

Avoid the use of physical restraint in medically ill or elderly patients with agitation and aggressive behaviors

Physical restraint involves the use of physical or mechanical devices to restrain movement. The use of physical restraints in medically ill patients, especially the elderly, is associated with loss of function; can result in greater personal and financial costs for individuals, families, and society; and may result in severe injury, worsening disability, frailty, and death.[5–7] Because of the high risks associated with physical restraint, new rules have emerged over the past decade prohibiting routine use of physical restraints in patients. Documentation is required to demonstrate that alternatives to restraint were used or attempted.[8,9] New rules issued by the Centers for Medicare and Medicaid Services (CMS)[9] mandate that health care workers who employ physical restraints and seclusion when treating patients must undergo new, rigorous training to ensure the appropriateness of the treatment and to protect patients' rights. The new rules, published in the *Federal Register* (December 8, 2006), limit episodes of physical restraint to up to 4 hours for adults; they may be applied for emergency use only if needed to ensure the patient's safety when less restrictive interventions have been ineffective.[10] Restraints may not be used for discipline or staff convenience or as a substitute for active treatment.

Common pitfalls

Medications with anticholinergic effects, including mid-potency DRAs, should be avoided in patients with hallucinogen intoxication, as the drugs may be mixed with anticholinergic compounds. Close monitoring is necessary when managing patients with agitation, and psychiatric consultation is usually required. Many patients with agitation require inpatient care.

Although pharmacological intervention for severe agitation and/or aggressive behaviors is commonly provided as needed, prolonged conditions may be better controlled by use of scheduled dosing, as indicated in the first vignette. However, the potential benefit of antipsychotic medications for controlling agitation and aggressive behaviors must be carefully weighed against the potential harm, and unnecessary prolonged use should be discouraged should the clinical condition permit.

Physical restraint is discouraged. Frequent assessment to ensure the patient's safety, such as vital signs and circulation distal to the restraint, is required during the restraint phase.

References

1. Leutmezer F, Podreka I, Asenbaum S, et al. Postictal psychosis in temporal lobe epilepsy. *Epilepsia*. 2003;44(4):582–590.

2. Stoudemire A, Fogel BS, Gulley LR. Psychopharmacology in the medical ill: an update. In: Stoudemire A, Fogel BS (eds.), *Medical Psychiatric Practice*. Washington, DC: American Psychiatric Press; 1991:129.

3. Van der Bijl P, Roelofse JA. Disinhibitory reactions to benzodiazepines: a review. *J Oral Maxillofac Surg*. 1991;5:519.

4. Wise MG, Rundell JM. *Concise Guide to Consultation Psychiatry*. Washington, DC: American Psychiatric Press; 1988:21.

5. Mohr WK, Petti TA, Mohr BD. Adverse effects associated with physical restraint. *Can J Psychiatry*. 2003;48:330–337.

6. Sullivan-Marx EM. Delirium and physical restraint in the hospitalized elderly. *J Nursing Scholarship*. 1994;26:295–300.

7. Weiss EM, Megan K, Blint DF, Altimari D. Deadly restraint: a *Hartford Courant* investigative report. *Hartford Courant*. 1998; October 11–15.

8. Gross G, Mitchell B, Hayes A. *Restraint and Seclusion—Overview of Federal Laws and Policies* (2003). Available at: http://www.hogg.utexas.edu/docs/062207_FederalLaws%20.PPT. Accessed July 1, 2008.

9. Department of Health and Human Services. Centers for Medicare & Medicaid Services Web site. Available at: www.cms.gov. Accessed December 19, 2007.

10. *Federal Register: Rules and Regulations*. 2006;71(236).

Chapter 12

The patient with psychotic symptoms

Glen L. Xiong

Clinical scenario

A 20-year-old man is brought in by his mother for insomnia and worsening anxiety. He reports that he has been having chest pain for over 2 months. His responses to questions are slow and terse. After much effort, you gather that he is "nervous" because he is afraid of demons, but he will not elaborate further. His mother reports that the patient has been staying in his room over the past 3 months. About 8 months ago, he quit his job as a waiter because of stress from classes. Later he stopped attending community college. The mother reports that he has not been eating, bathing, or changing his clothes regularly. His room is in complete disarray. She has seen him talking to himself at times.

Approach to history-taking and workup

Unique features of patients with psychotic or thought disorders and skills used during assessment

The patient may present with anxiety, depression, suspiciousness, social withdrawal, or somatic symptoms rather than overt psychotic symptoms.[1] Because of perceptual and expressive deficits, speech and thoughts are often marked by a paucity of content and are prone to derail. For this reason, taking histories from and interviewing psychotic patients is often disjointed and lacks coherence (or linearity). Proceed slowly, with frequent pauses and clarifications, rather than jumping from question to question. Anticipatory guidance—explaining to the patient clearly about the therapeutic intention of the provider—may assuage the patient's perception of possible threats. Reassuring statements such as, "I'm here to help and I'm glad you are trying the best you can with the answers" are helpful.

Confrontation or rationalization about the presence of delusions or hallucinations should be avoided. Empathize with the patient's distress rather than confirming or challenging a particular symptom or belief. Accompanying family members or familiar others may serve as a safety net.

Collateral information is critical, as the patient's story is often incomplete.[2] While family members may confuse psychosis with depression, anxiety, insomnia, and "strange" behavior, they are also able to objectively report on the patient's general functioning (such as dropping out of school, not caring for hygiene) and any overt delusions or hallucinations.

A longitudinal developmental and social history can help the physician decide whether the patient is suffering from a chronic persistent illness such as schizophrenia or an episodic phenomenon such as a mood-related psychosis. A substance use history should be obtained, though no amount of history is more definitive than a urine drug screen, which should be obtained in all cases of psychosis.

Physical symptoms may be the primary presentation, either as part of an underlying delusion or as misinterpretation of a physical ailment. Therefore, physical symptoms need to be evaluated carefully. The acuity and duration of the symptoms can be used to dictate the workup. A risk–benefit ratio for invasive procedures should be assessed individually. For example, if the patient in the case scenario is convinced that he is having a heart attack and has no risk factors, an intensive cardiac workup could be deferred, especially if the symptoms have been occurring for several months. An electrocardiogram, however, could be both reassuring and medically indicated.

Ensuring safety of patient and others

An acutely psychotic patient may be agitated or violent. Safety should be the physician's number one priority. Conduct the interview in a room where an exit is readily available for the patient and the provider. Avoid sitting directly between the patient and the door, but also ensure a direct route of escape if the situation necessitates one. Some questions are useful for confimation of safety, such as, "Would it be O.K. if I continue to ask you more questions? Do you feel safe talking to me here?" Most nonpsychiatric facilities are not equipped to care for a patient with acutely agitated psychosis; therefore, enlist help from security personnel as indicated.

Differential diagnosis

More often than not, a patient who "hears voices" or "sees things" is given a diagnosis of schizophrenia, but not all cases of hallucinations are secondary to schizophrenia. To meet the *DSM-IV-TR* diagnostic criteria for schizophrenia, a patient must have two of the following symptoms: (1) delusions, (2) hallucinations, (3) disorganized speech (frequent derailment or incoherence), (4) disorganized or catatonic behavior, and/or (5) negative symptoms (affective flattening, alogia [poverty of speech], or avolition).[3] If the delusions are bizarre or if hallucinations consist of a voice commenting on the person's behavior or thoughts or two or more voices talking with each other, then either of these symptoms alone is sufficient. Other criteria include impairment of socio-occupational functioning and a duration of 6 months or greater of continuous signs of disturbance. Exclusion of mood, substance, and medical disorders as etiologic is mandatory for a diagnosis of schizophrenia.[4] For the medical provider, it is initially more important to determine the presence and cause of psychosis (using terms such as psychotic disorder NOS) because diagnostic boundaries of the various disorders often overlap, and symptoms may change over time.

Table 12.1 lists common conditions that should be included in the differential diagnosis of psychosis. One common challenge in the diagnosis of schizophrenia is distinguishing it from a mood-related psychosis or a substance-induced psychosis.[5] A patient with a mood-related psychosis often (but not always) presents with mood-congruent psychotic themes. For example, a patient with mania usually presents with grandiose delusions. In patients with isolated hallucinations and delusions without any prominent interpersonal deficits, the diagnosis of malingering should be considered, and neuropsychological testing may be requested (refer to Chapter 19, "The Patient with Unusual Presentations," and Chapter 23, "Neurocognitive and Psychological Assessment"). If a patient's symptoms correlate well with the initiation of a medication (or illicit substance), a drug-induced psychosis is likely. However, in all cases of first-episode psychosis, a drug screen is warranted. In the population with chronic disease, especially older patients, an episode of psychosis may be related to a change in medical conditions, such as CNS infection or other accident, systemic infection, metabolic

Table 12.1 Differential diagnosis of psychosis

Psychiatric disorders

- Schizophrenia
- Schizophreniform disorder
- Schizoaffective disorder
- Bipolar disorder, with psychotic features
- Major depressive disorder, with psychotic features
- Psychotic disorder, not otherwise specified
- Delusional disorder
- Brief reactive psychosis
- Borderline personality disorder (with transient psychosis)
- Post-traumatic stress disorder
- Mental retardation
- Malingering
- Delusion of parasitosis (monosymptomatic hypochondriacal psychosis)
- Dissociative disorder

Medical disorders

- Drug-induced psychosis (opiates, steroids, antibiotics, chemotherapy)
- Dementia (Alzheimer's, vascular, mixed)
- Delirium
- Seizure disorder
- CNS infection (HIV, syphilis, herpes encephalitis)
- Systemic vasculitides (lupus, CNS vasculitis)
- Brain metastases
- Parkinson's disease
- Huntington's disease
- Hypo-/hyperthyroidism
- Electrolytes (hypercalcemia, uremia)
- Nutrition (thiamine, vitamin B_{12} deficiencies)

abnormalities, or even an isolated urinary tract infection (refer to Chapter 13, "The Patient with Confusion or Memory Problems").

To rule out potentially reversible or organic causes of psychosis, a complete medical evaluation is required. Delirium should be the default diagnosis in acutely ill medical-surgical settings until a complete medical evaluation and medication review have been conducted and are negative. The presence of psychotic symptoms in an elderly patient without acute medical conditions calls for screening for dementia.[6] Basic laboratory studies for the workup of psychosis are similar to those for delirium (refer to Chapter 5, "Psychiatric Emergencies," and Chapter 13, "The Patient with Confusion or Memory Problems"). These include but are not limited to basic chemistries, calcium, complete blood count, thyroid panel, syphilis serology, HIV antibody, vitamin B_{12}, folate, possibly thiamine, and brain imaging (as indicated). Sedimentation rate and ANA tests may be considered if a connective tissue disease or autoimmune disease process is suspected. A urine drug screen is mandatory in the setting of new psychosis. More specific investigations such as lumbar puncture and further rheumatological studies should be individually considered. Table 12.2 summarizes an initial workup of a patient who presents with psychosis.

Treatment strategies

The treatment of psychotic disorders is dictated by etiology. For patients whose psychosis is rooted in medical causes or medications, antipsychotics are used for symptom control while underlying issues are addressed. Common symptoms improved by antipsychotic medications include agitation, violent urges or behavior, and significant distress with or without behaviors resulting from psychotic symptoms. Managing these secondary psychoses requires resolution of the underlying etiology.

When a drug-induced psychosis is suspected, discontinue the agent, and the patient may not need any antipsychotic medication. However,

Table 12.2 Workup of psychosis

- Obtain urine toxicology screen for drug of abuse (mandatory)
- Assess for delirium (altered level of consciousness)
- Review medications carefully and discontinue medications that may cause psychosis (opiates, anticholinergics, benzodiazepines, antibiotics, immunological agents)
- Consider toxin exposure (lead poisoning, heavy metals)
- Check for nutritional depletion (vitamin B_{12}, folate, thiamine)
- Look for concurrent mood disorder (depressive or manic episode)
- Rule out dementia
- Evaluate for medical causes of psychosis (e.g., HIV and other CNS infections, traumatic brain injury, seizure disorder, multiple sclerosis)
- *Recommended laboratory studies*: TSH, syphilis serology, vitamin B_{12}, folate, complete blood count, electrolytes, calcium
- *Other laboratory studies to consider*: HIV, thiamine, ESR, CRP, ANA, lumbar puncture
- Brain imaging

certain medications may have to be tapered, such as opiates or steroids. Addition of antipsychotic medication for symptom control is reasonable in such situations, especially when a medication cannot be discontinued, such as steroid treatment in autoimmune diseases or immunomodulators in post–organ transplant medications.

Antipsychotic use in patients with dementia has recently received much scrutiny due to increased cerebrovascular events and mortality, and this off-label use is controversial[7] (refer to Chapter 4, "Overview of Psychopharmacologic Therapies").

Because the long-term use of antipsychotics may be associated with long-term motor, cognitive, and metabolic side effects, antipsychotic use for drug-induced or any secondary psychosis should be discontinued as soon as possible or maintained at the lowest possible dose.

In cases of chronic persistent mental illness (e.g., schizophrenia), it is prudent to refer patients to mental health agencies for integrated medical and psychosocial treatments when possible. These patients will often require "wraparound" services that include housing, transportation, group therapy, job training, and application for disability, in addition to medication. In rural communities, however, patients with persistent psychosis due to schizophrenia or bipolar disorder are often treated by primary care providers. Such providers will need to develop an ongoing collaborative relationship and close communication with a mental health team.[8] Consultation via telepsychiatry is an emerging model for rural providers.[9] Education and psychosocial support may be obtained from consumer groups such as the National Alliance on Mental Illness (NAMI) and other community resources. In such cases, when a primary care provider has to prescribe an antipsychotic for a schizophrenic patient, the rule of thumb is to try not to alter medication or dosages unless a psychiatric consultation is obtained, unless severe or life-threatening side effects dictate more rapid action.

Patients with delusions of parasitosis (a variant of hypochondriasis),[10] psychosis secondary to depressive and anxiety disorder, delirium- and dementia-related psychosis, and other psychosis due to a medical condition are most likely encountered in nonpsychiatric medical settings. Some of these medical patients may require indefinite antipsychotic treatment. Therefore, it is important to be familiar with antipsychotic pharmacology and to seek collaboration/consultation whenever possible. When an antipsychotic is indicated, a second-generation (or "atypical") antipsychotic is usually selected, based on the patient's underlying medical comorbidities, cost, and potential adverse effects (refer to Chapter 4, "Overview of Psychopharmacologic Therapies").

Common pitfalls

Psychotic disorders are commonly encountered in nonpsychiatric settings. Not all patients with delusions or hallucinations have schizophrenia, and patients with schizophrenia may not necessarily present with (or even have) delusions or hallucinations. Many mental health facilities do not have the technical expertise or laboratory or imaging studies available to detect occult medical disorders. Therefore, a new diagnosis of psychosis should always be scrutinized and warrants careful workup, including a urine drug screen, before committing a patient to a psychiatric institution. Finally, a patient's longitudinal history should be carefully reviewed, as psychosis may be secondary to mood disorder, personality disorder, delirium, or dementia.

References

1. Ferran E, Barron C, Chen T. Psychosis. *West J Med.* 2002;176(4):363–366.

2. Keks N, Blashki G. The acutely psychotic patient. *Aust Fam Physician.* 2006; 35(3):90–94.

3. American Psychiatric Association. *Diagnostic and Statistical Manual of Mental Disorders, 4th Edition, Text Revision.* Washington, DC: American Psychiatric Association; 2000.

4. Lehman AF, Lieberman JA, Dixon LB, et al.; American Psychiatric Association. Practice guideline for the treatment of patients with schizophrenia, second edition. *Am J Psychiatry.* 2004;161(S2):1–56.

5. Citrome L. Differential diagnosis of psychosis: a brief guide for the primary care physician. *Postgrad Med.* 1989;85(4):273–280.

6. Battista MA, Emes R, Ahles S. Psychosis in late life: evaluation and management of disorder in primary care. *Geriatrics.* 2005;60:26–33.

7. Gill SS, Bronskill SE, Normand SLT, et al. Antipsychotic drug use and mortality in older adults with dementia. *Ann Intern Med.* 2007;146:775–786.

8. Verdoux H, Cougnard A, Grolleau S, Besson R, Delcroix F. How do general practitioners manage subjects with early schizophrenia and collaborate with mental health professionals? A postal survey in South-Western France. *Soc Psychiatry Psychiatry Epidemiol.* 2005;40(11):892–898.

9. O'Reilly R, Bishop J, Maddox K, Hutchinson L, Fisman M, Takhar J. Is telepsychiatry equivalent to face-to-face psychiatry? Results from a randomized controlled equivalence trial. *Psych Services.* 2007;58(6):836–843.

10. Bhatia MS, Jagawat T, Choudhary S. Delusional parasitosis: a clinical profile. *Int J Psychiatry Med.* 2003;30(1):83–91.

Chapter 13

The patient with confusion or memory problems

Sarah K. Rivelli

Clinical scenario

Mrs. G, a 76-year-old woman with COPD, CHF, diabetes, and a history of transient ischemic attacks, is brought to your clinic by her daughter for follow-up after hospitalization for a fall. Her daughter explains that the patient was "talking out of her head" and "yelling and screaming" during the hospitalization. Luckily, Mrs. G sustained no injuries from her fall. The daughter recalls that her mother was treated for a urinary tract infection during the inpatient stay. The daughter asks for your opinion about what happened to her mother and wonders, "Is she demented now?"

Approach to history-taking

Patients presenting with confusion are difficult to assess without additional information from family or friends, particularly because the patient may be unaware of deficits or inaccurate in reporting. It is important to use collateral information to illuminate the patient's functioning at home, ability to manage affairs, and ability to care for himself or herself. Evaluate the patient's ability to perform activities of daily living (ADLs), such as bathing, dressing, walking, using the toilet, and feeding himself or herself. Ask about the patient's instrumental activities of daily living (IADLs)—ability to cook, shop, clean, pay bills, make appointments, and use the telephone.

Examine the time course of the cognitive decline to determine whether it occurred precipitously or insidiously, and gradually or stepwise. Obtain past and present psychiatric and medical history; this may reveal risk factors for confusional states or certain types of dementia. Careful review of medications and any recent medication changes may point to a cause of cognitive dysfunction.

Dementia diagnosis

Dementia is not a normal result of aging, though its prevalence increases with age. The prevalence of dementia in people at age 60 is 1%, but by age 85 it is about 50%.[1] Dementia should be considered when a patient has repeatedly missed appointments, missed paying bills, has trouble handling paperwork or following directions, appears confused about medication or treatment instructions, or has difficulty making medical decisions.[2] Patients with dementia are frequently (though not always) unaware of their memory problems. Additional history may include recent motor vehicle accidents, falls, increased ER visits, delirium, stroke, unexplained weight loss, or a change in functional status. A decline in self-care, such as grooming and hygiene, may also indicate dementia.[2] Social skills are often preserved in many forms of dementia, and thus a patient may appear appropriate during a short office visit.

The diagnosis of dementia includes memory impairment and at least one other cognitive impairment: agnosia, aphasia, apraxia, or a disturbance in executive functioning. Functional impairment must be present for a diagnosis of dementia.[3]

There are several subtypes of dementia. Understanding the nature and extent of the type of dementia may inform the prognosis and treatment. Alzheimer's disease (AD), the most common dementia, accounts for at least half of cases. Vascular and frontotemporal dementias account for another 15% each. Many patients have "mixed dementia," with features of both AD and vascular dementia. Dementia with Lewy bodies (DLB) accounts for 5% to 10% of dementias.[4] Table 13.1 lists unique features of each subtype of dementia.

Reversible dementia is quite rare: only 1.5% of cases of mild to moderate dementia are fully reversible.[3] Causes of reversible dementia include hypothyroidism and vitamin B_{12} deficiency. Normal-pressure hydrocephalus (NPH) leads to ataxic gait, urinary incontinence, and dementia. Even after treatment of NPH by high-volume lumbar puncture or placement of a ventriculo-peritoneal shunt, however, significant cognitive deficits may remain.

The Mini-Mental State Examination (MMSE)[4] is the most commonly used and studied screening test for dementia. It can be administered in less than 10 minutes. It is 71% to 92% sensitive and 56% to 96% specific for dementia, with a median positive likelihood ratio (LR) of 6.3 (95% confidence interval

Table 13.1 Unique features of dementia subtypes				
	Alzheimer	**Vascular**	**Frontotemporal**	**Lewy body**
Onset	Gradual	Acute/subacute	Earlier	Variable
Course	Progressive	Stepwise	Rapidly progressive	Variable
Prominent symptoms	Forgetting, particularly short-term memory loss	Focal neurological deficits, evidence of CVA or small-vessel ischemic changes on imaging	Deficits in planning, impulsivity, personality change, language difficulties	Visual hallucinations, fluctuating cognition, falls, parkinsonism

[CI] 3.4 to 47) and negative median LR of 0.19 (95% CI 0.06 to 0.37).[5] The MMSE tests multiple domains of cognition, though assessment of executive function is lacking. The most common thresholds for an abnormal result are 23 or 24, though age and education may contribute to the interpretation of results. The MMSE may not be sensitive enough to capture mild dementia in highly educated subjects, and there may be false negatives in this setting. False positives may occur among those with lower education and in non-white subjects.[5]

The Mini-Cog is a shorter screening test for dementia; it takes only 2 to 4 minutes to complete. It has been validated in general practice and appears less sensitive to language and cultural differences and educational bias than the MMSE.[6] Patients are asked to remember three unrelated words, then to draw a clock, and then to recall the three words. Scoring is simple: patients are initially classified by the number of words they recall. Those who recall all three words are classified as nondemented, while those who recall none of the three words are classified as probably demented. Patients who recall one or two words are classified according to their performance on the clock-drawing test, with an abnormal clock leading to classification as probably demented. The clock is considered normal if all numbers are present and in correct sequence and the hands are placed at the right time. This test had a sensitivity of 76% and specificity of 89% in a multiethnic community sample of older subjects[7] and had even higher sensitivity and specificity in clinical samples of older subjects with memory complaints. Patients who screen positive for possible or probable dementia can be referred for further cognitive evaluation (refer to Chapter 23, "Neurocognitive and Psychological Assessment").

Differential diagnosis

Delirium and depression are necessary differentials (Table 13.2).

Depression

Depression can lead to "pseudodementia"—cognitive deficits due to lack of motivation and self-efficacy. In contrast to demented patients, patients with depression and memory loss are aware of their deficits and give up easily on formal mental status evaluation. Performance on testing may improve with encouragement. Such patients can be distinguished from those with dementia by the presence of neurovegetative symptoms, such as lack of appetite, and mood symptoms, such as sadness. Neurocognitive testing may clarify the etiology of cognitive complaints (refer to Chapter 23, "Neurocognitive and Psychological Assessment"). With successful treatment of depression, complaints of memory loss diminish and scores on formal mental status tests improve. However, pseudodementia may be an early sign of "true" dementia.[8]

Delirium

Delirium, also called altered mental status, acute confusional state, or encephalopathy, is characterized by an acute onset of altered consciousness

Table 13.2 Differential diagnosis of selected syndromes

	Dementia	Delirium	Depression	Psychosis
Onset	Gradual	Acute	Varies	Varies
Course	Progressive	Fluctuates	Variable	Variable
Sensorium	Altered, clouded	Clear	Clear	Clear
Memory	Impaired	Impaired	Largely conserved	Conserved
Attention	Intact	Impaired	Intact	Impaired
Psychomotor	May be agitated, can be retarded in late stages	Hypoactive or hyperactive	Retarded	May be agitated
Hallucinations	Visual or auditory	Visual, tactile, auditory	Auditory	Auditory
Delusions	Usually persecutory	Often paranoid	Classically mood congruent	Complex, paranoid
Mood	May be apathetic	Labile	Sad, dysphoric	Varies

that fluctuates and is generally reversible.[3] Impaired attention that waxes and wanes over a short time is the hallmark of delirium; patients may appear easily distracted and require prompting to cooperate with the interview. Thought process may be disorganized. Delusions may occur and may be inspired by external stimuli, such as an intravenous catheter. Perceptual disturbances may range from illusions to frank auditory, tactile, or visual hallucinations. Patients without a prior history of psychosis who present with visual hallucinations are more likely to have delirium than a primary psychotic disorder. Language may be vague and perseverative. Patients may have dysphoric, euphoric, or labile affect and thus may appear significantly manic or depressed.

Patients with delirium may be hyperactive and agitated and may harm themselves. Patients may also present with hypoactivity, apathy, withdrawal, and paucity of speech. Sleep disturbances include reversal of the day/night cycle with frequent naps and insomnia.

The Confusion Assessment Method is a valid, reliable screening tool for the detection of delirium (Table 13.3).[9]

Memory impairment and disorientation may be present in both delirium and dementia, and amnesia alone is not sufficient for either diagnosis. History may reveal risk factors, medical conditions, or medications that might cause dementia or delirium. Dementia itself is also a risk factor for delirium.

Evaluation of the patient with confusion

A thorough medical workup, including a physical examination, should be undertaken to seek underlying causes of delirium or reversible causes of dementia. For example, asterixis may suggest the presence of hepatic or

Table 13.3 Confusion Assessment Method (CAM)

1. Acute onset of changes or fluctuations in the course of mental status—Is there evidence of an acute change in mental status from the patient's baseline? Did the abnormal behavior fluctuate during the day—that is, tend to come and go, or increase and decrease in severity?

2. Inattention—Did the patient have difficulty focusing attention—for example, being easily distractible or having difficulty keeping track of what was being said?

3. Disorganized thinking—Was the patient's thinking disorganized or incoherent, such as rambling or irrelevant conversation, unclear or illogical flow of ideas, or unpredictable switching from subject to subject?

4. Altered level of consciousness—Overall, how would you rate this patient's level of consciousness?

   Normal = alert

   Hyperalert = vigilant

   Drowsy, easily aroused = lethargic

   Difficult to arouse = stupor

   Unarousable = coma

   Screen is positive for delirium if 1 and 2 are present plus either 3 or 4.

Reprinted with permission from Inouye SK, van Dyck CH, Alessi CA, Balkin S, Siegal AP, Horwitz RI. Clarifying confusion: the Confusion Assessment Method. A new method for detection of delirium. *Ann Intern Med.* 1990;113(12):941–948.

uremic encephalopathy. Tremor and visual hallucinations may be seen in alcohol or sedative withdrawal. Myoclonus is seen in many toxic-metabolic syndromes, including drug toxicities such as lithium toxicity. The presence of altered mental status, hyperreflexia, diarrhea, and flushing is consistent with serotonin syndrome. Altered mental status, rigidity, and fever in the setting of antipsychotic medication use is concerning for neuroleptic malignant syndrome (refer to Chapter 5, "Psychiatric Emergencies").

Common underlying causes of delirium include the following:

- Intracranial causes (cerebrovascular events, subdural hematomas, tumors, encephalitis or meningitis)
- Systemic causes (metabolic derangements such as uremia, liver failure, hypoxemia, and hypoglycemia)
- Vitamin deficiencies and endocrinopathies (hypothyroidism, adrenal insufficiency, hypercortisolemia)
- Systemic infections (urinary tract infection, pneumonia, sepsis)
- Exogenous toxins (medications, drugs, especially anticholinergic agents)
- Withdrawal syndromes (alcohol and benzodiazepine withdrawal)
- Seizure, postictal state or nonconvulsive status epilepticus

Reversible causes of dementia traditionally include the following, though cognitive deficits may be only partially reversible:

- Vitamin B_{12} deficiency
- Hypothyroidism
- Neurosyphilis
- Normal-pressure hydrocephalus

Routine testing for apolipoprotein E ε4, which has been linked to AD, is not recommended, as many individuals homozygous for this allele will not develop AD.

Brain imaging should be performed for new-onset confusion or sudden cognitive impairment, particularly if focal neurologic signs are present. Noncontrast head CT is readily accessible and does not require prolonged cooperation from the patient. MRI may provide more detail of white matter disease and regional volume loss, such as smaller hippocampi in AD or decreased frontal lobe volume in frontotemporal dementia.

Electroencephalography (EEG) is useful for the evaluation of seizure or nonconvulsive status epilepticus, which can lead to the clouded sensorium seen in delirium. EEG shows diffuse slowing in delirium but is generally normal in mild to moderate dementia and psychiatric disorders. As dementia progresses, EEG shows increased slow wave activity and does not help discriminate the disorder from delirium.[10]

Treatment strategies

Reversible pathologies that may cause or contribute to cognitive impairment should be evaluated and treated. Therefore, it is important to seek and treat general medical conditions that may worsen cognitive function. Medications should be reviewed: anticholinergics should be discontinued, and sedatives tapered with a goal of discontinuation.

Dementia

Specific treatments for dementia are limited (refer to Chapter 4, "Overview of Psychopharmacologic Therapies"). The cholinesterase inhibitors donepezil, rivastigmine, and galantamine are approved for mild to moderate AD, while donepezil is also approved for severe AD, if patients can tolerate side effects and cost. There is some evidence of benefit in dementia associated with Parkinson's disease, DLB, and vascular dementia. Memantine is a noncompetitive NMDA receptor antagonist approved for treatment of moderate to severe AD. It is well tolerated, with modest benefits and few adverse effects. There is limited evidence that it benefits vascular dementia.

NSAIDs and estrogen have shown a lack of efficacy and safety in placebo-controlled trials in AD and are not recommended.

Behavioral disturbances in dementia

Agitation, aggression, hallucinations, and delusions are common in patients with dementia and are a common reason for placement in nursing homes.[11] When such symptoms occur, careful evaluation for medical, environmental, and psychosocial problems should first be undertaken. Nonpharmacological intervention with redirection, reassurance, and correction of any unmet needs is indicated. If symptoms cause significant distress or danger, antipsychotics may be prescribed, but careful evaluation of the risks and benefits is necessary (refer to Chapter 11, "The Patient with Agitated Symptoms"). There are no medications specifically approved for use in behavioral disturbances associated with dementia. Randomized controlled trials do not consistently support the use of antipsychotics for psychosis, agitation, and behavioral symptoms,[12,13] and these agents are associated with a significantly increased risk of mortality in this setting and carry a boxed warning. First- and second-generation antipsychotics appear to carry a similar risk of mortality in demented patients.[14] Benzodiazepines should be avoided due to the risk of impaired cognition, delirium, and falls.

Given the limited efficacy of medications in the treatment of dementia, psychosocial approaches, such as the following, should be used:

- Education of patient and family
- Frequent reorientation
- Reassurance
- Safety measures: minimize wandering, caution against driving
- Legal issues: plan for patient's eventual incapacity (advance directives, power of attorney, will and testament) (refer to Chapter 20, "The Patient Who Refuses Care")
- Caregiver support (support groups, respite care)
- Recreational therapy and stimulation (art therapy, music therapy, pet therapy)

Delirium

The main treatment approach in delirium is the search for the underlying cause(s) as described above. The following supportive measures may reduce the severity and duration of delirium:

- Reorientation
- Reassurance
- Identification and correction of sensory impairments (hearing aid, glasses)
- Sleep hygiene
- Low-stimulation environment
- Adequate physical activity (ambulation, gentle exercise)

Antipsychotics have been insufficiently studied for the treatment of delirium. The current practice is to use them for symptoms causing significant distress or danger after careful evaluation of the risks and benefits (refer to Chapter 11, "The Patient with Agitated Symptoms"). If antipsychotics are employed, the dose and duration should be minimized as much as possible.

Common pitfalls

Early diagnosis of dementia may allow the patient and family to complete advance directives and discuss end-of-life planning with the patient. Dementia is generally underdiagnosed in primary care, and many providers do not perform routine screening. Delirium and dementia are likely to co-occur in the elderly. Collateral information from friends and family can help determine if a patient is at his or her baseline. Psychosocial approaches are often overlooked despite limited evidence for pharmacological treatments for dementia and delirium.

References

1. Boustani M, Peterson B, Hanson L, Harris R, Lohr K. Screening for dementia in primary care: a summary of the evidence for the U.S. Preventive Task Force. *Ann Intern Med.* 2003;138(11):927–937.

2. Lawhorne L. Approaches to the office care of the older adult and the specter of dementia. *Prim Care Clin Office Pract.* 2005;32:599–618.

3. American Psychiatric Association. *Diagnostic and Statistical Manual of Mental Disorders, 4th ed., Text Revision.* Washington, DC: American Psychiatric Association; 2000.

4. Folstein MF, Folstein SE, McHugh PR. Mini-Mental State. A practical method for grading the cognitive state of patients for the clinician. *J Psychiatr Res.* 1975;12(3):189–198.

5. Holsinger T, Deveau J, Boustani M, Williams JW Jr. Does this patient have dementia? *JAMA.* 2007;297:2391–2404.

6. Borson S, Scanlan J, Brush M, et al. The Mini-Cog: a cognitive "vital signs" measure for dementia screening in multi-lingual elderly. *Int J Geriatr Psychiatry.* 2000;15:1021–1027.

7. Borson S, Scanlan JM, Chen P, et al. The Mini-Cog as a screen for dementia: validation in a population-based sample. *J Am Geriatr Soc.* 2003;51:1451–1454.

8. Brown WA. Pseudodementia: issues in diagnosis. *Appl Neurol.* 2005;1:40–42.

9. Inouye SK, van Dyck CH, Alesi CA, et al. Clarifying the confusion: the Confusion Assessment Method. A new method for detection of delirium. *Ann Intern Med.* 1990;113(12):941–948.

10. Smith SJM. EEG in neurological conditions other that epilepsy: when does it help, what does it add? *J Neurol Neurosurg Psychiatry.* 2005;76(Suppl II):ii8–ii12.

11. Yaffe K, Fox P, Newcomer R, et al. Patient and caregiver characteristics and nursing home placement in patients with dementia. *J Am Med Assoc.* 2002;287:2090–2097.

12. Schneider LS, Dagerman KS, Insel P. Efficacy and adverse effects of atypical antipsychotics for dementia: meta-analysis of randomized, placebo-controlled trials. *Am J Geriatr Psychiatry.* 2006;14:191–210.

13. Schneider LS, Tariot PN, Dagerman KS, et al. Effectiveness of atypical antipsychotic drugs in patients with Alzheimer's disease. *N Engl J Med.* 2006;355(15):1525–1538.

14. Wang PS, Schneeweiss SS, Avorn J, et al. Risk of death in elderly users of conventional vs. atypical antipsychotic medications. *N Engl J Med.* 2005;353:2335–2341.

Chapter 14

The patient with multiple physical complaints

Gregory Lunceford

Clinical scenario

A 28-year-old female graduate student presents to the acute care clinic with left hand numbness and left lower extremity weakness. Her symptoms began a week ago and have been increasing in severity. She decided to come in for medical attention today because she is unable to work on her dissertation project due to her symptoms. She was released from the hospital 10 days ago after an evaluation for new-onset seizures. During that hospitalization, she had an MRI, EEG, and blood work, all of which were negative. She is accompanied by her younger sister, who is concerned because their mother had a stroke 5 years ago and can't move her left side well. The patient also complains of poor energy and poor concentration. Over the past 5 days, she has spent most of her time in bed.

Background

Patients with medically unexplained symptoms (MUS) create a dilemma for the health care provider. There is always the fear of missing an organic illness and thereby not being of good service to the patient. These patients tend to seek more attention and emotional support, causing some physicians to feel pressured.[1] Caregivers have been characterized as being critical by these patients, particularly when caregivers are encouraging them to be less dependent.[2] Patients with MUS use resources at a high rate. They are prone to frequent medical visits, unnecessary tests, and unnecessary medical procedures. They are more likely to be unemployed and classified as disabled.[3]

For the purposes of this chapter, patients with MUS have been divided into two categories, the somatoform disorders (Table 14.1)[4] and functional syndromes (Table 14.2). For treatment purposes, the somatoform disorders can be further classified by distinguishing those with similarity to obsessive-compulsive disorder, specifically by separating out hypochondriasis and body dysmorphic disorder.

There are many functional syndromes; the four best described are fibromyalgia, irritable bowel syndrome, chronic fatigue syndrome, and non-ulcer dyspepsia. They are mentioned here because although they are well-described syndromes, their pathophysiology remains unknown.

Table 14.1 Somatoform disorders

Name of disorder	Differential features
Somatization disorder*	Multiple and recurrent physical complaints over several years
	Symptoms usually begin before age 30
Conversion disorder	One or more symptoms or deficits affect a voluntary motor or sensory function
	Symptoms suggest a neurological or general medical condition
Somatic pain disorder*	Pain in one or more anatomical locations
Hypochondriasis*	Preoccupation or idea with fears that one has a serious disease
	Based on misinterpretation of bodily symptoms
Body dysmorphic syndrome*	Preoccupation with an imagined defect in appearance or markedly excessive concern regarding slight physical anomaly
Factitious disorders*†	Conscious and voluntary production of physical or mental signs and symptoms (refer to Chapter 19, "The Patient with Unusual Presentations")

* To establish a diagnosis, those conditions must cause impairment in social or occupational function or in other important areas.

† Factitious disorder was previously labeled Munchausen's disorder/Munchausen's by proxy.

Source: American Psychiatric Association. Diagnostic and Statistical Manual of Mental Disorders, 4th ed., Text Revision. Washington, DC: American Psychiatric Association; 2000.

Table 14.2 Functional syndromes

Name of syndrome	Differential features*
Irritable bowel syndrome	Abdominal pain or discomfort and changes of bowel habits that are chronic and recurrent
Chronic fatigue syndrome	Severe chronic fatigue lasting 6 months or longer accompanied by four or more of the following: memory impairment, sore throat, tender lymph nodes, muscle pain, multiple joint pains without erythema or swelling, headache, unrefreshing sleep, post-exertional malaise
Fibromyalgia	Chronic widespread pain and exaggerated tactile pain response, usually accompanied by fatigue, poor sleep, functional bowel symptoms, cognitive dysfunction, anxiety, or depression
Non-ulcer dyspepsia	Persistent, recurrent upper abdominal discomfort, usually accompanied by nausea, emesis, early satiety, postprandial fullness, and abdominal bloating

* None of these conditions is explained by any abnormalities seen on routine clinical testing.

Evaluation

Patients with MUS present to a variety of clinical settings (e.g., the office, acute care clinics, emergency rooms). Their presentation may seem odd or atypical, immediately raising clinical suspicion. They may have an unusual affect or bizarre behavior. Many times, however, nothing may seem out of the ordinary early on.

History

Careful history-taking is critical in patients with MUS. They often present with a recurrent set of symptom complexes. It is important to nail down the chronology, character, location, and intensity of symptoms. Patients may refine their symptoms consciously and subconsciously with subsequent interviews, obscuring the appearance of a non-organic disorder. Documenting key historical data for subsequent providers is essential, particularly in the hospital setting, where many consultants can become involved.

Data collection

Often, patients with MUS have had many previous workups. Get all previous evaluations (e.g., lab tests, radiographic studies, pathology reports). Document when patients are evasive or guarded about disclosing their medical records. If they bring records with them, remember that patients with factitious disorders may be selective in terms of the documents they bring, bringing data that support their symptoms and omitting contradictory information. Hypochondriacal patients may be obsessively focused on positive studies and thereby omit the negative ones. Get collateral information from family and friends when possible and ask about the use of sedatives and analgesics, which may be excessive. Inquire about work status and activity level, which often do not correlate with physical findings—patients with MUS often function at an unusually low level.

Personal history

Getting at the psychiatric or psychological components is the major issue. It takes clinical skill to initiate this area of investigation without offending or upsetting the patient. Patients may take this line of questioning to mean that their medical complaints are not being taken seriously. Educate patients about the fact that stress and anxiety can cause a number of physical symptoms and can contribute to the development of a number of conditions.[4] If the patient is unreceptive at this point, it may be useful to point out that a number of tests and studies have been done without result, and if we are to be comprehensive, all aspects of treatment should be employed with an open mind. Reassure the patient that this line of investigation does not mean that he or she is being perceived as "crazy" or "unstable." Ask about stressful life events and try to correlate them with symptoms chronologically. Rule out anniversary reactions. Investigate physical and sexual abuse, particularly in childhood.[5]

Evaluation of anxiety and depression

Depression is common in patients with MUS. Depression itself has a variety of physical manifestations. Patients with fibromyalgia, non-ulcer dyspepsia, irritable bowel syndrome, and chronic fatigue syndrome suffer from depression at a higher rate than patients with similar conditions of known organic etiology.[6] Some argue that depression and anxiety describe functional disorders in patients with MUS better than the somatization disorders, particularly in patients presenting to the primary care setting.[6]

Treatment

In general, there are relatively few treatments for MUS. Evidence-based treatment modalities are lacking. There are data to support the psychiatric consultation letter, cognitive-behavioral therapy, and certain pharmacologic interventions.

Psychiatric consultation letter

Randomized, controlled studies have shown the psychiatric consultation to improve physical function and reduce the utilization of medical resources.[7] The letter includes the following points:

1. Establish the primary care physician as the patient's main and (if possible) only physician.
2. Set up regularly scheduled appointments every 4 to 6 weeks.
3. Keep outpatient visits brief.
4. Perform at least a partial physical exam each visit directed at the organ system of complaint.
5. Understand the symptoms as emotional communication rather than the harbinger of new disease.
6. Look for signs of disease rather than being symptom-focused.
7. Avoid diagnostic tests, laboratory evaluations, and operative procedures unless clearly indicated.
8. Set a goal of referring at least selected patients to psychiatric treatment.

Cognitive-behavioral therapy

Randomized, controlled trials have shown that cognitive-behavioral therapy (CBT) reduces symptoms and health care utilization. CBT is based on the principle that human thoughts generate human emotions, and our emotions can have an impact on health. In the case of patients with MUS, CBT focuses on reducing physical distress and somatic preoccupation through the following[8]:

1. Relaxation techniques—relaxation therapy is incorporated into everyday life and in response to physical discomfort.
2. Behavioral management—patients are taught to optimize their vocational, social, and self-care activities.
3. Cognitive restructuring—patients are taught to monitor their thoughts and emotions and how they trigger physical symptoms.
4. Emotional identification—patients are taught to identify "illness behaving."
5. Emotional regulation—patients are taught to address emotions that lead to "illness behaving."
6. Interpersonal skills training—patients are taught assertiveness training, which reduces suppressed emotion.

CBT is best when performed by trained therapists. Patients with MUS are often reluctant to pursue psychotherapy early on. There is evidence that some cognitive therapy interventions can be conducted well by the primary care physician and other primary care practitioners.[9,10]

Pharmacologic interventions

Hypochondriasis and body dysmorphic syndrome (BDS) have characteristics of obsessive-compulsive disorders (OCDs) and have been shown to respond well to treatments for OCDs. As with OCD, SSRIs and clomipramine have improved the treatment of hypochondriasis and BDS substantially. Data support the use of clomipramine, fluvoxamine, fluoxetine, and citalopram for the treatment of hypochondriasis. A randomized, controlled trial has shown efficacy for fluoxetine in the treatment of BDS.[11] The SSRIs seem to carry the most robust response, followed by the MAO inhibitors and lastly the tricyclic antidepressants.

There are no randomized, controlled trials showing efficacy of medications for somatization disorder, though some open-label studies have shown efficacy for SSRIs.

Other treatment issues

Sleep disorders are common in patients with MUS (both somatization and functional disorders). In many cases, referral for a formal sleep study is indicated (refer to Chapter 15, "The Patient with Disordered Sleep"). Addressing issues of sleep hygiene can also promote well-being. Patients with MUS tend to be chronically symptomatic; therefore, it is advisable to avoid hypnotic agents with tolerance and addiction potential. Consider a sedating antidepressant followed by a non-benzodiazepine sedative.

In the case of functional disorders, each has specific treatment options that will not be addressed in detail. For the purposes of this chapter, it is important to point out that the treatment of depressive disorders and anxiety disorders is essential. Data show that these disorders have strong ties to major depression and anxiety disorders.[5]

Common pitfalls

1. Avoid unnecessary procedures and interventions.
2. Beware of the potential for abuse of prescription analgesics and sedatives.
3. Be alert for patients with factitious disorders (refer to Chapter 19, "The Patient with Unusual Presentations").

Useful resources

deGruy F, Crider J, Hashimi DK, Dickinson P, Mullins HC, Troncale J. Somatization disorder in a university hospital. *J Fam Practice*. 1990;25:579–584.

Fallon B. Pharmacotherapy of somatoform disorders. *J Psychosom Res*. 2004; 56:455–460

Hinson VK, Haren WB. Psychogenic movement disorders. *Lancet Neurol.* 2006; 5:695–700.

Kroenke K. Somatoform disorders and recent diagnostic controversies. *Psychiatric Clin North Am.* 2007;30:593–619.

McDermott BE, Feldman MD. Malingering in the medical setting. *Psychiatr Clin North Am.* 2007;30:645–662.

Smith RC, Gardiner JC, Lyles JS, et al. Exploration of DSM-IV criteria in primary care patients with medically unexplained symptoms. *Psychosom Med.* 2005;65:123–129.

References

1. Salmon P, Ring A, Humphris GM, Dowrick CF. What do general practice patients want when they present medically unexplained symptoms, and why do their doctors feel pressurized? *J Psychosom Res.* 2005;59:255–262.

2. Salmon P, Phil D, Wissow L, et al. Doctors' responses to patients with medically unexplained symptoms who seek emotional support: criticism or confrontation? *Gen Hosp Psychiatry.* 2007;29:454–460.

3. Escobar JI, Swartz M, Rubio-Stipec M, Manu P. Medically unexplained symptoms: distribution, risk factors and comorbidity. In: Kirmayer LJ, Robbins JM, eds. *Current Concepts of Somatization: Research and Clinical Perspectives.* Washington, DC: American Psychiatric Press; 1991:63–78.

4. American Psychiatric Association. *Diagnostic and Statistical Manual of Mental Disorders, 4th ed., Text Revision.* Washington, DC: American Psychiatric Association; 2000.

5. Katon WJ, Walker EA. Medically unexplained symptoms in primary care. *J Clin Psychiatry.* 1998;59(supplement 20):15–21.

6. Henningsen P, Zimmermann T, Sattel H. Medically unexplained physical symptoms, anxiety and depression: a meta-analytic review. *Psychosom Med.* 2003:65:528–533.

7. Smith RG, Rost K, Kashner M. A trial of the effect of a standardized psychiatric consultation on health outcomes and costs in somatizing patients. *Arch Gen Psychiatry.* 1995:52:238–243.

8. Woolfolk RL, Allen LA, Tiu JE. New directions in the treatment of somatization. *Psychiatric Clin North Am.* 2007;30:621–644.

9. Smith RC, Lein C, Collins C, et al. Treating patients with medically unexplained symptoms in primary care. *J Gen Intern Med.* 2003;18:478–489.

10. Escobar JI, Gara MA, Diaz-Martinez AM, et al. Effectiveness of a time-limited cognitive behavior therapy type intervention among primary care patients with medically unexplained symptoms. *Ann Family Med.* 2007;5:328–335.

11. Phillips KA, Albertini RS, Rasmussen SA. A randomized placebo-controlled trial of fluoxetine in body dysmorphic disorder. *Arch Gen Psychiatry.* 2002;59(4):381–388.

Chapter 15

The patient with disordered sleep

Xavier Preud'homme

Clinical scenario

Ms. R is a 40-year-old woman in generally good health who presents for her annual primary care visit with Dr. X. During the visit, Ms. R complains of difficulty falling asleep and maintaining sleep. She does not meet criteria for depressive or anxiety disorder, and there are no acute health or social stressors that she can relate to her difficulties sleeping. She asks Dr. X for the latest sleep aid she has seen on commercials and gives him a toll-free number to call so she can have a free trial prescription.

Background

The American Academy of Sleep Medicine (AASM) practice parameters cumulatively offer a large body of evidence-based guidelines, as well as an algorithmic approach to diagnosing and managing common sleep complaints. In brief, the simplest and most effective method for sorting out sleep complaints is to group them into three distinct categories, which are listed here in order of decreasing prevalence:

1. Disorders of initiation and/or maintenance of sleep (DIMS)
2. Disorders of excessive daytime sleepiness (DOES)
3. Other disorders, such as the parasomnias (abnormal sleep events) and the circadian rhythm disorders (misalignment between desired and actual sleep period)

Box 15.1 lists common abbreviations used to describe the sleep disorders.

History-taking

The best ways to identify the causes of sleep complaints are a careful sleep history (Table 15.1),[1] a sleep log (diary), and, for some patients, overnight polysomnography (PSG). Figure 15.1 shows the relationship between the three aforementioned classifications. A sleep log/diary is helpful for diagnosing DIMS and circadian disorders, whereas polysomnography (in association with audio-video recording) is helpful to elucidate DOES and the

Box 15.1 Abbreviations

AASM	American Academy of Sleep Medicine
AHI	Apnea hypopnea index
AHS	Alveolar hypoventilation syndrome
APAP	Automatic self-adjusting positive airway pressure
ASPD	Advanced sleep phase disorder
BiPAP	Bilevel positive airway pressure
CPAP	Continuous positive airway pressure
CSA	Central sleep apnea syndrome
CSR	Cheyne-Stokes respiration
DIMS	Disorders of initiation and/or maintenance of sleep
DOES	Disorders of excessive daytime sleepiness
DSPD	Delayed sleep phase disorder
MSLT	Mean sleep latency test
NREM	Non-rapid eye movement
OSA	Obstructive sleep apnea syndrome
PAP	Positive airway pressure
PLMD	Periodic leg movement disorder
PSG	Polysomnography
REM sleep	Rapid eye movement
RERA	Respiratory effort–related arousal
RLS	Restless leg syndrome
SBRD	Sleep-related breathing disorder

Table 15.1 Important aspects of sleep history and rationale

Important to elicit . . .	In order to detect . . .
Symptoms of heightened arousal	Hyperarousal and hyperactivity to stressors are common characteristics of patients with insomnia, who show increased metabolic rate (suggesting a strong physiological component to this disorder).
Symptoms or a history of depression or anxiety or other major psychopathology	There is a high prevalence of psychiatric disorders in patients presenting with insomnia.
Symptoms of restless legs syndrome or periodic limb movement disorder	Both conditions are prevalent in patients complaining of insomnia but can also be the presenting complaint for further underlying medical or neurological problems (e.g., iron deficiency, parkinsonism, peripheral neuropathy).
Sleep/wake schedule disorders	History is the key here, and several weeks of sleep logs can serve as a confirmatory test.
Snoring and other symptoms of sleep apnea	Sleep apnea is a common cause of excessive daytime sleepiness and also of interrupted nighttime sleep, which when presented as the primary complaint can lead to a diagnosis of insomnia without polysomnography (and treatment for obstructive sleep apnea syndrome would differ from treatment of primary insomnia).
Symptoms or a history of drug or alcohol abuse	Drugs and alcohol use have long-lasting effects on sleep.

Table 15.1 *continued*	
Important to elicit . . .	In order to detect . . .
Current medication use (including OTC medications)	Medications are common causes of insomnia complaints and daytime sedation and can worsen apneas or periodic leg movements.

Source: Chesson A Jr, Hartse K, Anderson WM, et al. Practice parameters for the evaluation of chronic insomnia. *Sleep.* 2000;23(2):1–5.

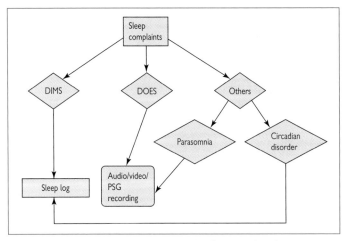

Figure 15.1 Algorithm for sleep complaints: classification and work-up.

parasomnias. *Daytime sleepiness*, as opposed to fatigue, is the determining feature distinguishing DOES from DIMS. To assess daytime sleepiness, a self-report assessment such as the Epworth Sleepiness Scale[2] quantifies the ease with which one would fall asleep across eight different situations (e.g., while resting, watching TV, driving). Each answer is rated from 0 (never) through 3 (high probability of falling asleep), for a total possible score of 24. The cut-off for pathological excessive daytime sleepiness is 10. In one study, the following mean scores were reported by distinct populations: controls (5.9), insomniacs (2.2), sleep apnea (11.7), residents (14.6), and narcolepsy (17.5).[3]

Even though sleep hygiene (Table 15.2) is part of the therapeutic plan, it is worth having those instructions in mind when reviewing the sleep history to better target the intervention to a particular patient.

Differential diagnosis and management strategies

Disorders of initiation or maintenance of sleep (DIMS)

Insomnia is the most common sleep complaint: 33% of the general population reports insomnia symptoms, one-third of those with insomnia complain of daytime consequences, and one-fifth meet formal *DSM-IV*[4]

Table 15.2 Sleep hygiene instructions

1. Keep the same schedule for going to bed and getting up, 7 days a week.
2. Keep your bedroom at a comfortable temperature and free of light and noise.
3. Eat regular meals but none for at least 2 hours prior to bedtime. Avoid drinking excessive liquids in the evening.
4. Avoid alcohol (in particular when presenting with disorders of excessive daytime sleepiness) and all caffeine products (especially when presenting with disorders of initiation or maintenance of sleep).
5. Consider smoking cessation.
6. Exercise regularly, preferably in the later part of the afternoon, but never later than 6 or 7 p.m.
7. Use the bedroom only for sleeping and sexual activity. Do not work in your bedroom or watch TV. Work out your problems and worries prior to bedtime.
8. When the presenting complaint is DIMS or circadian disorder, avoid naps during the day and, at night, limit time in bed to time asleep.
9. If unable to fall asleep within 15 to 30 minutes, leave the bedroom and try again later after engaging in nonstimulating activity under dim light (less than 150 lux).

Source: Stepanski EJ, Wyatt JK. Use of sleep hygiene and the treatment of insomnia. *Sleep Med Rev.* 2003;7(3):215–225.

Table 15.3 Simplifying the diagnosis of insomnia

Subjective complaint of difficulties . . .	Associated with:
Falling asleep	Marked distress
or	or
Staying asleep	Significant daytime impairment
or	
Nonrestorative sleep	

Source: *Diagnostic and Statistical Manual of Mental Disorders, Fourth Edition,* Text Revision (DSM-IV-TR). Washington, DC: American Psychiatric Association; 2000; Chesson A Jr, Hartse K, Anderson WM, et al. Practice parameters for the evaluation of chronic insomnia. *Sleep.* 2000;23(2):1–5.

diagnostic criteria for a disorder (Table 15.3).[5] Insomnia is more common among women, middle-aged and elderly people, shift workers, and patients with medical and/or psychiatric disorders. A good sleep history is fundamental to the assessment of insomnia complaints and often will serve as the primary diagnostic tool. It is also helpful in differentiating between primary and secondary insomnia, the latter being more recently referred to as comorbid insomnia. Polysomnography (PSG) is not indicated in the workup of transient insomnia, routine chronic insomnia, or comorbid insomnia secondary to psychiatric disorders, but PSG should be considered "when a sleep-related breathing disorder or periodic limb movement disorder is suspected, initial diagnosis is uncertain, treatment fails, or precipitous arousals occur with violent or injurious behavior."[6]

A recent review of the National Institutes of Health statement regarding the management of chronic insomnia in adults[7] led Buysse[8] to suggest the following:

- Most cases of chronic insomnia coexist with other medical or psychiatric conditions, yet *the treatment of comorbid insomnia should not be withheld pending the treatment of these other conditions.* For example, for a depressed patient with complaints of insomnia, it is important to address both up front.

- When choosing medications for the treatment of insomnia (refer to Chapter 4, "Overview of Psychopharmacologic Therapies"), selective benzodiazepine receptor agonists (e.g., zolpidem, zaleplon, eszopiclone) are the safest and are effective, and should therefore be used as first-line agents. It is also a good idea to use slow-release formulations when prescribing medications for maintenance in insomnia.
- The following five behavioral treatments are empirically supported by evidence cited in the AASM practice parameters:[5]
  1. Stimulus control therapy
  2. Relaxation
  3. Paradoxical intention
  4. Sleep restriction
  5. Cognitive-behavioral therapy
- These behavioral and psychological treatments may be best accomplished by referral to a sleep specialist.

Disorders of excessive daytime sleepiness (DOES)

Sleep deprivation is statistically the most common cause of excessive daytime sleepiness. Sleep-related breathing disorders (SRBDs) and the periodic leg movements disorder (PLMD) are other common contributors to daytime sleepiness. Narcolepsy is a rare cause of daytime sleepiness and should be included in the differential diagnosis; however, patients with suspected narcolepsy should be referred for specialist evaluation.

Sleep-related breathing disorders

Abnormal breathing in sleep includes snoring, hypopneas, apneas, and respiratory effort–related arousals (RERAs). Because such events may be present in normal sleepers, SRBDs are syndromes defined by the high frequency of these events producing either symptoms or adverse health outcomes.

The gold standard for the evaluation of SRBDs is PSG.[5] However, because of internight variability, the sensitivity of one night of PSG to detect a pathological index of apneas and hypopneas (Apnea-Hypopnea Index ≥5/h of sleep) is only 60% to 88%.

Some clinical prediction models, such as one based on upper airway and body measurements,[9] achieve a very high sensitivity. Nevertheless, in practice a full PSG remains a necessary step and will be needed to determine response to treatment. Also, many insurance companies will not reimburse treatments for disorders diagnosed based on clinical prediction models or portable monitoring.[1]

The standard treatment approach of the SRBDs, which include obstructive sleep apnea syndrome (OSA), central sleep apnea syndrome (CSA), Cheyne-Stokes respiration (CSR), and alveolar hypoventilation syndrome (AHS), is to use positive airway pressure (PAP), especially when increased respiratory efforts to breathe against relative or absolute airway obstruction (OSA) have been identified.[10] At present PAP devices are promoted in three forms: continuous (CPAP), bilevel (BiPAP), and automatic self-adjusting (APAP). Though a full-night attended study performed in a sleep laboratory is the preferred approach to determine the optimal positive pressure for maintaining airway patency, the split-night diagnostic-titration study remains acceptable.

CPAP is the first-line treatment of moderate to severe OSA, but there is also some evidence for its usefulness in mild OSA in reducing self-reported sleepiness, in improving quality of life, in lowering blood pressure in hypertensive patients (as adjunctive therapy), and probably in lowering resistance to antidepressants in patients with comorbid depression.[10] BiPAP should be considered, as it lowers the pressure during the expiratory phase of the respiratory cycle, in patients requiring high pressure, those who experience difficulties exhaling against a fixed pressure, or patients with coexisting restrictive lung diseases or hypoventilation syndrome complicated by daytime hypercapnia.[10] Side effects of CPAP and BiPAP are negligible and reversible.

APAP should not be used in the initial determination of treatment response; its use should also be restricted to the management of patients presenting with loud OSA (since the PAP auto adjustment relies on noise) without any other cardiopulmonary complications.[11]

When managing SRBDs it is important to closely monitor the adequate use of the PAP as well as compliance. Systematic educational programs and the addition of a heated humidifier have been shown to increase utilization.

Special considerations: Cardiac conditions and populations at risk for SBRDs
SBRD should be ruled out in symptomatic patients with congestive heart failure (CHF), as in one study it was present in 75% and 50% of men and women, respectively.[9] Male gender, age greater than 60 years, and presence of atrial fibrillation were significantly predictive of CSA, whereas BMI > 35 was significantly predictive of OSA. SBRDs (principally CSA) were also frequently found in patients with coronary artery disease (CAD) to the extent that the slightest suspicion of sleep apnea in these patients should prompt referral for PSG. Likewise, PSG to rule out OSA should always follow a finding of unexplained right ventricular failure. Furthermore, 40% of patients undergoing placement of an automatic internal cardioverter-defibrillator met criteria for SBRDs, more often CSA than OSA, the former being associated with a worse overall prognosis. Patients with recurrent atrial fibrillation after cardioversion, tachyarrhythmia, or bradyarrhythmia should also be carefully screened for SBRDs. Finally, SBRDs are a risk factor for strokes and, unless corrected, have an adverse impact on survival and prognosis.[9]

Periodic leg movement disorder
Periodic leg movement disorder (PLMD) is characterized by sleep that is interrupted by repetitive movements primarily involving the legs, with subsequent sleep complaints associated with this excess of movements. It is

picked up by PSG with 82% sensitivity and 100% specificity.[12] PLMD is also found in 80% to 90% of patients complaining of restless legs syndrome (RLS), an unpleasant urge to move the legs. Both PLMD and RLS respond well to dopaminergic agonists (the lowest effective dose is recommended), though seeking underlying causes and treating them, particularly when iron disorders are found, is a priority in order to avoid the unpleasant side effects of dopaminergic agents (sleepiness and [rarely] sleep attacks, insomnia, GI disturbance, fluid retention, and occasionally worsening of the target symptoms).

Narcolepsy

Narcolepsy, characterized by brief, irresistible daytime sleep episodes with or without catalepsy, sleep paralysis, and sleep hallucinations, occurs equally in men and women and has its onset in the early to mid-20s in almost 90% of those affected. A PSG followed by a mean sleep latency test (MSLT) is required to confirm the diagnosis of narcolepsy,[13] and the patient should be referred to a specialist for both diagnosis and management.

Common pitfalls

When a parasomnia, characterized as an abnormal event occurring during sleep (i.e., REM sleep behavior disorder), is suspected, a PSG with audio and video recording is indicated to make the diagnosis, while its management will likely be initiated by a sleep specialist.

Patients with circadian rhythm disorders may be initially diagnosed with DIMS (when focusing on their inability to fall or remain asleep) or DOES (when focusing on their increased daytime sleepiness). A good sleep history will point to exogenous factors (shift work, jet lag) as well as to endogenous factors, especially in the case of advanced and delayed sleep phase disorders (ASPD, DSPD). Sleep diaries spanning several weeks are also useful; for patients with refractory symptoms, it is a good idea to consider referral to a sleep clinic for confirmation by actigraphy and for management.[14]

References

1. Chesson AL, Berry RB, Pack A. Practice parameters for the use of portable monitoring devices in the investigation of suspected obstructive sleep apnea in adults. A joint project sponsored by the American Academy of Sleep Medicine, the American Thoracic Society, and the American College of Chest Physicians. *Sleep.* 2003;26(7):907–913.

2. Johns MW. A new method for measuring daytime sleepiness: the Epworth Sleepiness Scale. *Sleep.* 1991;14:540–545.

3. Papp KK, Stoller EP, Sage P, et al. The effects of sleep loss and fatigue on resident-physicians: a multi-institutional mixed-method study. *Acad Med.* 2004;79:394–406.

4. *Diagnostic and Statistical Manual of Mental Disorders, Fourth Edition, Text Revision* (DSM-IV-TR). Washington, DC: American Psychiatric Association; 2000.

5. Morin CM, Bootzin RR, Buysse DJ, et al. Psychological and behavioral treatment of insomnia: update of the recent evidence (1998–2004). *Sleep.* 2006;29(11):1398–1414.

6. Littner M, Hirshkowitz M, Kramer M, et al. for the Practice Committee of the American Academy of Sleep Medicine. Practice parameters for using polysomnography to evaluate insomnia: an update for 2002. *Sleep.* 2003;26(6):754–760.

7. National Institutes of Health. State of the Science Conference Statement. Manifestation and management of chronic insomnia in adults. *Sleep.* 2005;28(9):1045–1053.

8. Buysse DJ. Insomnia state of the science: an evolutionary, evidence-based assessment. *Sleep.* 2005;28(9):1045–1046.

9. Kushida CA, Littner MR, Morgenthaler T, et al. Practice parameters for the indications for polysomnography and related procedures: an update for 2005. *Sleep.* 2005;28(4):499–521.

10. Kushida CA, Littner MR, Hirshkowitz M, et al. Practice parameters for the use of continuous and bilevel positive airway pressure devices to treat adult patients with sleep-related breathing disorders. *Sleep.* 2006;29(3):375–380.

11. Littner M, Hirshkowitz M, Davila D, et al. for the Practice Committee of the American Academy of Sleep Medicine. Practice parameters for the use of auto-titrating continuous positive airway pressure devices for titrating pressures and treating adult patients with obstructive sleep apnea syndrome. *Sleep.* 2002;25(2):143–147.

12. Hening WA, Allen RP, Early CJ, et al. for the Practice Committee of the American Academy of Sleep Medicine. A review by the Restless Legs Syndrome Task Force of the Standards of Practice Committee of the American Academy of Sleep Medicine. An update on the dopaminergic treatment of restless legs syndrome and periodic limb movement disorder. *Sleep.* 2004;27(3):560–583.

13. Littner MR, Kushida C, Wise M, et al. for the Practice Committee of the American Academy of Sleep Medicine. Standards of Practice Committee of the American Academy of Sleep Medicine. Practice parameters for clinical use of the multiple sleep latency test and the maintenance of wakefulness test. *Sleep.* 2005;28(1):113–121.

14. Morgenthaler TI, Lee-Chiong T, Alessi C, et al. Standards of Practice Committee of the AASM. Practice parameters for the clinical evaluation and treatment of circadian rhythm sleep disorders. *Sleep.* 2007;30(11):1445–1459.

Chapter 16

The patient with low weight or abnormal eating behaviors

Wei Jiang

Clinical scenario

A 20-year-old female college student in her junior year is referred to the student health clinic by her coach, who is concerned about the student's low weight. The patient is reluctant to be seen, stating that she does not need to gain weight. She says she is "as fat as a cow." She is a cross-country runner on the varsity team and has no past medical history. She admits having occasional chest "fluttering" and lightheadedness. She says her weight has been in the high 80s since age 16. Because her running has not been as fast as she would like, she has worked on losing more weight recently. She admits that she is distressed by the compulsion she feels to count the calories she consumes daily. She denies taking any medication or other substances. On physical exam, her skin is pale, her hair is dry, her heart rate is 48, and her blood pressure is 84/54. Her weight is 79 pounds, and she stands 5'6". She says she has not had her period since she graduated from high school. Although she denies behaviors of binging or purging, the exam reveals erosion of the enamel of the front teeth and scars on the knuckles of the left hand.

Background

Perhaps in association with the United States' cultural obsession with models and actors displaying an unattainable level of thinness, anorexia nervosa (AN) has become an increasingly prevalent problem. The 2005 Youth Risk Behavior Survey revealed that 32% of adolescent girls believed they were overweight and 61% were attempting to lose weight.[1] In the 30 days before questioning, 6% of adolescent girls reported they had tried vomiting or had taken laxatives to help control their weight. Many clinicians believe that increased numbers of eating-disordered patients are presenting to their practices. An estimated 1 to 2 million women in the United States meet the criteria for bulimia nervosa (BN) as defined in the *DSM-IV-TR*;[2] 500,000 women meet the diagnostic criteria for AN.[3] Many more have disordered eating but do not fulfill the criteria for AN or BN, meeting criteria for ED NOS. There are two peaks of the onset of AN, at ages 14 and 18, though patients may present from late childhood through adulthood.

Although commonly thought to be a female problem, males experience eating disorders too, with a ratio of female to male of between 10:1 and 20:1. The prevalence of eating disorders in males may be rising: more males sought treatment for eating disorders in the 1990s than in the 1980s.[4]

Making a proper diagnosis and identifying complications

The *DSM-IV-TR*[2] classifications of eating disorders include AN, BN, and ED NOS. Because AN is a potentially lethal disorder, health care providers must ensure early identification and proper treatment. While patients with BN or ED NOS may be well managed in the primary care setting by primary care providers, AN should be managed by a specialized eating disorder treatment team. In any event, medical complications of eating disorders require attention from primary care providers and other medical specialists.

Table 16.1 lists the characteristics that distinguish AN from BN. Patients with ED NOS may have certain features of each but do not meet the full criteria for either one.

Screening tools

There are two short screening instruments (5 questions each), the SCOFF and the ESP questionnaires, that may assist the clinician in identifying patients who need further evaluation (Tables 16.2 and 16.3). Responding "yes" to two or more questions on the SCOFF was initially associated with a sensitivity of 100% and specificity of 87.5% for the diagnosis of an eating disorder.[5] However, a subsequent report comparing ESP and SCOFF revealed the sensitivity and specificity of SCOFF to be lower (78% and

Table 16.1 Features differentiating anorexia nervosa (AN) and bulimia nervosa (BN)

Features	AN	BN
Weight	Low, <85% expected	Normal or higher
Intense fear of increasing weight	Yes	No
Disturbance in weight and/or body size	Yes	No
Menses	Absent	Present
Eating behaviors	Restriction May binge and/or purge	Binge and/or purge
Malnutrition symptoms	Present	Absent
Attitude toward treatment	Opposes	Accepts
Respond to SSRI	No	Yes

88%, respectively), while two abnormal responses to ESP had a sensitivity of 100% and specificity of 71%.[6] Further validation of these instruments is needed in broader populations.

Physical examination

The following components of the physical examination are important in evaluating a patient with an eating disorder:

- Weight and height for Body Mass Index (BMI)
- Temperature and supine/standing heart rate, blood pressure for hypothermia and orthostatic hypotension
- Skin and extremity for dryness, bruising, lanugo (abnormal fine hair growth on extremities), or Russell's sign (scars on knuckles of the fingers resulting from inducing vomiting)
- Cardiac examination for bradycardia, arrhythmia, or mitral valve prolapse
- Facial examination for parotid gland hypertrophy, erosion of the enamel of the anterior teeth from vomiting

Laboratory assessment

Patients with eating disorders should be screened with the following laboratory studies:

- Complete blood count for anemia or other hematologic abnormalities

Table 16.2 SCOFF questionnaire

- Do you make yourself **S**ick because you feel uncomfortably full?
- Do you worry you have lost **C**ontrol over how much you eat?
- Have you recently lost more than **O**ne stone (14 lbs or 6.35 kg) in a 3-month period?
- Do you believe yourself to be **F**at when others say you are too thin?
- Would you say that **F**ood dominates your life?

One point for every "yes"; a score of >2 indicates a likely case of anorexia nervosa or bulimia.

Reprinted with permission from Morgan JF, Reid F, Lacey JH. The SCOFF questionnaire: assessment of a new screening tool for eating disorders. BMJ. 1999;319(7223):1467–1468. *BMJ* Publishing Group Ltd.

Table 16.3 ESP questionnaire

The ESP has 5 questions to screen for eating disorders:

- Are you satisfied with your eating patterns? (No is abnormal)
- Do you ever eat in secret? (Yes is abnormal)
- Does your weight affect the way you feel about yourself? (Yes is abnormal)
- Have any members of your family suffered with an eating disorder? (Yes is abnormal)
- Do you currently suffer with or have you ever suffered in the past with an eating disorder? (Yes is abnormal)

Reprinted with permission from Cotton M-A, Ball C, Robinson P. Four simple questions can help screen for eating disorders. *J Gen Intern Med*. 2003;18(1):53-56. Blackwell Publishing.

- Glucose, electrolytes, calcium, magnesium, phosphorous, blood urea nitrogen, and creatinine for dehydration or purging, need for admission, or refeeding syndrome
- B-hCG to exclude pregnancy as causative for amenorrhea; thyroid function tests as well as measurement of serum prolactin and follicle-stimulating hormone can be obtained to rule out amenorrhea due to prolactinoma, hyperthyroidism, hypothyroidism, or ovarian failure
- Urinalysis to assess specific gravity—AN patients may water-load to falsely elevate weight (an unexplained low specific gravity may be due to water-loading)
- EKG for patients with bradycardia or arrhythmia
- Lipase level (elevation suggests purging or vomiting)
- Urine drug screen is indicated when use of substances or stimulants to reduce weight is suspected
- Stool laxative screen when abuse is suspected

Complications

Many medical complications can occur with chronic starvation or persistent purging:

- Electrolyte abnormalities, particularly hypokalemia and metabolic alkalosis, in patients who purge by vomiting, laxative abuse, or diuretic abuse
- Osteopenia or osteoporosis
- Growth delay
- Cardiac arrhythmia or cardiac failure
- Cognitive changes
- Difficulty in psychological functioning
- Gastrointestinal dysfunction such as slowed motility and symptoms of nausea or bloating
- Endocrinologic changes from AN may include low serum LH and FSH concentrations, "sick euthyroid syndrome" with increased levels of reverse T3, low serum dehydroepiandrosterone (DHEA) and insulin-like growth factor-I (IGF-I), and increased serum cortisol and growth hormone concentrations
- Dental erosion and enlarged salivary glands in patients with BN
- Infertility

Differential diagnosis

The differential diagnosis for weight loss or chronic vomiting can be extensive. The following illnesses need to be considered and ruled out in most AN patients:

- New-onset diabetes mellitus may present with severe weight loss
- Adrenal insufficiency may present with weight loss, orthostasis, and depression
- Primary depression with anorexia must be differentiated from AN

- Inflammatory bowel disease, celiac disease, or other gastrointestinal diseases must be considered
- Abdominal masses can cause chronic vomiting
- Central nervous system lesions can cause vomiting, appetite suppression, and a depressed affect

Clinical management

As noted in Table 16.1, the challenges in managing BN and AN are quite different.

Bulimia nervosa

Compared with AN, treatment of BN is more straightforward, with a high success rate. Cognitive-behavioral therapy (CBT) is the first-line treatment for BN[7] and is aimed at eliminating core features of BN as well as improving associated symptoms such as low self-esteem and depression. Long-term maintenance is better reached with CBT than antidepressant drugs. Given its success with BN patients, CBT also has been adapted for and found effective in patients with binge eating disorder.[7,8] Interpersonal therapy (IPT) may be considered if a patient does not respond to CBT.[9]

Fluoxetine is FDA-approved for treatment of BN based on effectiveness in several studies. A higher dose of fluoxetine resulted in greater improvement of BN symptoms.[7,10] Non-SSRI (selective serotonin reuptake inhibitor) antidepressants are also more effective than placebo at decreasing binging and vomiting in patients with BN. However, the better safety and side-effect profiles of the SSRIs make these drugs more attractive for first-line therapy. The antiepileptic agent topiramate and the selective serotonin antagonist ondansetron may be helpful in reducing binge and purge behaviors.

Anorexia nervosa

AN involves complex and challenging psychological issues and can have life-threatening medical consequences. Because patients frequently reject help and are chronically undernourished, the assessment and care of AN patients is often extremely difficult.

When encountering a patient with AN, appropriate triage is imperative. The patient may need urgent hospitalization, or perhaps referral to a specialized program (inpatient or outpatient) is appropriate. Conditions requiring urgent admission are potentially life-threatening, such as cardiac arrhythmia, severe electrolyte disturbance (hypokalemia, hyponatremia, hypophosphatemia) or dehydration, acute medical complications of malnutrition (e.g., syncope, seizures, cardiac failure, pancreatitis, acute renal failure), or acute psychiatric emergencies (e.g., suicidality with high-lethality plan or attempt, acute psychosis).

Patients with the conditions listed in Table 16.4 are best treated in a multidisciplinary program designated for eating disorder treatment with an inpatient setting or day program including attention to psychiatric, behavioral,

Table 16.4 Conditions benefiting from multidisciplinary care in an inpatient or day program setting

- Severe malnutrition (weight <75% of average body weight for age, sex, and height) with medical instability (significant bradycardia, hypotension, metabolic abnormality: glucose or electrolytes, dehydration, or evidence of organ compromise)
- Arrested growth and development
- Failure of outpatient treatment
- Acute food refusal
- Uncontrollable binging and purging
- Comorbid diagnosis that interferes with the treatment of eating disorders (e.g., severe depression, obsessive-compulsive disorder, severe family dysfunction)
- Weight <85% normal body weight or rapid decline with food refusal despite outpatient or partial hospitalization treatment
- Comorbid psychiatric conditions
- Poorly motivated patient needing assistance to eat or cooperative only in a highly structured environment

social, and general medical issues. Detailed methodology used by multidisciplinary eating disorder programs is beyond the scope of this book.

Summary

Patients with eating disorders, especially AN, are at high risk for severe and life-threatening medical as well as psychiatric comorbidities.

- Care for patients with AN can be highly challenging because of their lack of insight into their underlying illness and frequent refusal of care.
- AN is best managed by a multidisciplinary team involving nutritional rehabilitation, medical monitoring, and psychological treatment. Psychological treatment may include CBT, family therapy, or other psychological modalities. CBT emphasizes the relationship of thoughts and feelings to behavior and helps patients learn to recognize the thoughts and feelings that lead to disordered eating.
- For patients with BN, a combination of an antidepressant and psychotherapy[11] provides the best chance for remission.
- Patients with severe medical or psychological manifestations may require urgent hospitalization.

References

1. Eaton EK, Kann L, Kinchen S, et al. Youth risk behavior surveillance—United States, 2005. *MMWR Surveill Summ.* 2006;55:1.

2. *Diagnostic and Statistical Manual of Mental Disorders, Fourth Edition, Text Revision* (DSM-IV-TR). Washington, DC: American Psychiatric Association; 2000.

3. International Academy of Eating Disorders. *Position statement on equity in insurance coverage for eating disorders.* McLean, VA: Academy for Eating Disorders; 1997.

4. Braun DL, Sunday SR, Huang A, Halmi KA. More males seek treatment for eating disorders. *Int J Eat Disord.* 1999;25:415.

5. Morgan JF, Reid F, Lacey JH. The SCOFF questionnaire: assessment of a new screening tool for eating disorders. *BMJ.* 1999;319:1467.

6. Cotton M-A, Ball C, Robinson P. Four simple questions can help screen for eating disorders. *J Gen Intern Med.* 2003;18:53.

7. Wilson GT, Fairburn CG. Treatments for eating disorders. In: Nathan PE, Gorman JM (eds.), *A Guide to Treatments that Work.* New York: Oxford University Press; 1998:501.

8. Wilfley DE, Agras WS, Telch CF, et al. Group cognitive-behavioral therapy and group interpersonal psychotherapy for the nonpurging bulimic individual: a controlled comparison. *J Consult Clin Psychol.* 1993;61:296.

9. Fairburn CG, Norman PA, Welch SL, et al. A prospective study of outcome in bulimia nervosa and the long-term effects of three psychological treatments. *Arch Gen Psychiatry.* 1995;52:304.

10. Fluoxetine Bulimia Nervosa Collaborative Study Group. Fluoxetine in the treatment of bulimia nervosa. A multicenter, placebo-controlled, double-blind trial. *Arch Gen Psychiatry.* 1992;49:139.

11. Bacaltchuk J, Hay P, Trefiglio R. Antidepressants versus psychological treatments and their combination for bulimia nervosa. *Cochrane Database Syst Rev.* 2001;CD003385.

Chapter 17

The geriatric patient

Sarah K. Rivelli and Jane P. Gagliardi

Clinical scenario

Mrs. E, a 90-year-old woman, presents to the clinic for a routine visit. She lives at home with her husband, who is 93 and in poor health, and their daughter, who is very concerned about Mrs. E's month-long history of decreased appetite, decreased ambulation, and decreased interaction with family members. Mrs. E has a history of vascular dementia but has been independent in her activities of daily living until recently, when her daughter has had to help her bathe, brush her teeth, and get dressed. Her daughter is concerned that Mrs. E is becoming depressed due to her husband's failing health.

Background

The majority of elderly patients receive mental health care from their primary providers,[1] and there are unique issues to consider when treating them.

Approach to history-taking

Elderly patients commonly experience dementia, delirium, and depression. Substance use disorders may also be present and are easy to overlook. Evaluation of the patient's family and social situation is crucial. Establish rapport not only with the patient but also with family members to obtain collateral information and develop treatment plans.

Elderly patients are more likely to have multiple medical comorbidities that affect their functioning, quality of life, and mental status. Known and unknown medical problems may mount and contribute to a patient's affective and cognitive state. Sometimes even common problems such as a urinary tract infection or even constipation can worsen cognitive status. Keep these issues in mind when evaluating elderly patients.

Evaluate geriatric patients for the following:

- Cognitive status
  - Consciousness, orientation, memory, reasoning, language, visuospatial abilities
- Mood symptoms
  - Anhedonia, sadness

- Energy level
- Loss of appetite, weight loss
- Suicidality
  - Suicidality is **not** part of normal grieving and should prompt psychiatric referral
- Sleep
  - Insomnia is common in elderly patients and may be related to depression or dementia
- Living environment
- Elder abuse or neglect
- Social support and situation in case of end-of-life decision-making
  - Next of kin and/or health care power of attorney, trusted decision-maker
  - Guardianship status, if relevant
- Functional status
  - Activities of daily living (ADLs)—bathing, dressing, feeding
  - Instrumental activities of daily living (IADLs)—shopping, cooking, finances, complex activities
- Medical comorbidities
- Medication regimen
  - New or recently discontinued medications
  - Polypharmacy, drug interactions
  - Problems with adherence or medication errors

Important diagnostic considerations

A patient presenting with mood symptoms may actually be suffering the effects of cognitive impairment, which could be chronic, as with dementia, or more acute, as with delirium (refer to Chapter 13, "The Patient with Confusion or Memory Problems"). Nevertheless, geriatric patients with multiple medical problems and declining social support are at high risk for depression, increased health care costs, and completed suicide.[2] Major depressive disorder affects about 5% to 10% of older adults visiting their primary care provider and can be associated with worse outcomes from medical problems.[3–5]

Depression screening can be effectively carried out in elderly patients by using two questions contained in the Patient Health Questionnaire-2 (PHQ-2).[6] A positive screen can be followed by the Patient Health Questionnaire-9 (PHQ-9) to confirm the diagnosis of depression and to monitor symptom severity and response to treatment[7] (refer to Chapter 7, "The Patient with Depressive Symptoms").

Depressive symptoms may be seen in a variety of neurological diseases such as multiple sclerosis and Parkinson's disease. Both depression and dementia are common among patients with Parkinson disease; up to 25% may have major depression, while almost 30% meet criteria for dementia.[8,9] Post-stroke depression affects 25% to 50% of patients after stroke. Such patients may also present with cognitive decline.

Hypothyroidism is associated with depression, though depressive symptoms are unlikely to be fully explained by an elevated TSH alone; treating both the hormone deficiency and depression is warranted. Depression is more prevalent among patients with coronary artery disease, cancer, and many other medical conditions that are common in the elderly.[10]

Because neurovegetative symptoms of depression such as anorexia, weight loss, and fatigue can also be seen in a variety of medical illnesses, a thorough history and physical exam are warranted when such symptoms are present. Patients with depression should be evaluated for a history of mania, as the course and treatment of bipolar disorder vary from those of unipolar depression. Although rare, new-onset mania or psychosis without medical etiology may occur in elderly patients (refer to Chapter 4, "Overview of Psychopharmacologic Therapies," and Chapter 8, "The Patient with Manic Symptoms"). Assessment of suicidality is critical as depression in the elderly is associated with completed suicide, particularly among white men.

Cognitive impairment or reports of worsening memory may be a sign of dementia. Patients with dementia do not often self-report cognitive impairment and may be unaware of it. Deficits may be noted by concerned family members only once the patient experiences serious functional decline. Signs of cognitive impairment include missed appointments, difficulty understanding or remembering instructions, car accidents, or poor hygiene and grooming. Early detection may delay loss of independence and reduce family stress and burden.[11] Cognitive deficits may also represent "pseudo-dementia" related to depression, or delirium, which requires a medical workup (refer to Chapter 13, "The Patient with Confusion or Memory Problems").

Treatment strategies

Late-life depression

Establish safety by asking about suicidal thoughts or plans to end one's life (refer to Chapter 5, "Psychiatric Emergencies," and Chapter 6, "Suicide Risk Assessment"). The rate of death from suicide is highest in late life, and elderly white men are at greatest risk. Family members may need to be enlisted to remove weapons or access to medications.

Antidepressants are effective for the acute treatment of depression in the elderly.[12] Older tricyclic antidepressants (TCAs) and the newer selective serotonin reuptake inhibitors (SSRIs) and serotonin-norepinephrine reuptake inhibitors (SNRIs) have similar efficacy, but the newer agents are preferred due to their more benign side-effect profile (refer to Chapter 4, "Overview of Psychopharmacologic Therapies"). Long-term maintenance treatment with antidepressants can prevent recurrence of depression in the elderly. A combination of pharmacotherapy and psychotherapy provides the best results for late-life depression.[13]

Randomized, controlled trials have found that electroconvulsive therapy (ECT) is safe and effective in 60% to 80% of patients with severe late-life depression.[14] Expert consultation for evaluation for ECT is recommended, particularly for severe or psychotic affective states.

Education about depression and its symptoms and treatment helps reduce stigma and self-blame and promotes engagement in care. Sleep hygiene, including being active during the day and avoiding daytime sleep, helps improve mood and functioning (refer to Chapter 15, "The Patient with Disordered Sleep"). Counsel patients to avoid common over-the-counter sleep aids containing diphenhydramine, which impair cognition and are associated with delirium.

Psychotherapy is the preferred treatment modality among the elderly with depression,[15] yet patients are rarely referred. The greatest evidence favors cognitive therapy, behavioral therapy, and cognitive-behavioral therapy (CBT) for late-life depression.[12] Additional approaches supported by some evidence include problem-solving therapy, interpersonal therapy, and reminiscence therapy. There is also evidence for the benefit of exercise and in-home geriatric health evaluation and management in mild to moderate depression.[2] Be aware of available local mental health services to facilitate timely and appropriate referrals.

The primary care provider may have limited time to treat depression in an elderly patient with multiple competing health care needs. Collaborative care (a care manager working with the primary care provider to develop a treatment plan [medication and/or brief psychotherapy] in addition to patient tracking, education, and counseling) is a promising strategy, with twofold-higher effectiveness and improved functional outcomes when compared with usual care for geriatric depression.[16,17]

Dementia

Pharmacological treatments for dementia show only modest efficacy (refer to Chapter 4, "Overview of Psychopharmacologic Therapies," and Chapter 13, "The Patient with Confusion or Memory Problems"). Medication treatment for behavioral disturbances in dementia, such as agitation and psychosis, is controversial. Antipsychotics are frequently prescribed to treat such symptoms, but their use is limited by a significantly increased risk of death in this population.[18] It is important to assess patients with behavioral disturbances and cognitive impairment for medical comorbidities or environmental disturbances, prioritizing efforts to evaluate and treat pain, intercurrent illness, and delirium. Benzodiazepines are not recommended in the treatment of dementia as they worsen cognition, may cause behavioral disinhibition, and increase the risk of falls.

Common pitfalls

Stigma often leads patients not to seek care for their symptoms. Providers and patients alike frequently dismiss depressive symptoms as an inevitable part of aging, physical illness, or grief.

Specific cautions regarding medications in elderly patients are as follows:

- Pharmacokinetics
  - Geriatric patients have:
    - diminished hepatic and renal metabolism and excretion; and
    - reduced lean body mass and body water, with greater availability of water-soluble agents and decreased availability of fat-soluble agents.
- Pharmacodynamics: drug–drug interactions and polypharmacy are problematic.
- Adverse effects
  - Decreased autonomic homeostasis associated with aging contributes to increased risk for falls.
  - Medications that may cause orthostatic hypotension (such as alpha-blockers or antipsychotics) can be particularly dangerous in elderly patients.
  - Benzodiazepines are associated with increased risk for falls, worsening cognitive impairment, and possible disinhibiting effects in patients with cognitive disorders.
  - Antipsychotic medications have a few specific adverse effects:
    - Antipsychotics may increase prolactin levels and may contribute to osteoporosis.
    - When used to treat psychosis and agitation in dementia, antipsychotics are associated with a significantly higher rate of death. Second-generation antipsychotics have received a boxed warning; studies of first-generation antipsychotics have shown at least an equivalent risk.
    - SSRIs may be associated with an increased risk of osteoporosis; however, depression itself is implicated in the development of osteoporosis.
  - SSRIs are associated with an increased incidence of SIADH and clinically significant hyponatremia.
  - The routine use of TCAs is not recommended in elderly patients due to the risk for orthostatic hypotension, anticholinergic effects, and cardiac conduction abnormalities.
  - Lithium is renally cleared.
    - Elderly patients are at higher risk for lithium toxicity.
    - Maintenance lithium levels should be at the lower end of the therapeutic range in the elderly (0.5 to 0.6) and should be closely monitored.
    - Medications that decrease the renal clearance of lithium (ACE inhibitors, NSAIDs, diuretics) increase the risk of both renal insufficiency and lithium toxicity.

General recommendations

- "Start low and go slow" when titrating medications.
- Limit the number of medications prescribed.

- Emphasize non-pharmacological measures.
- Remember the importance of sleep hygiene.
- Emphasize the importance of exercise.
- Encourage pleasurable activities and stimulation.
- Solicit participation from family and support system.
- Provide education about mental health.
- Refer for psychotherapy, when available.

Useful resources

Patient information and education

Geriatric Mental Health: http://www.gmhfonline.org/gmhf/

IMPACT: http://impact-uw.org

Michigan Dementia Coalition: http://worriedaboutmemoryloss.com

Guidelines

Agency for Healthcare Research and Quality: http://www.ahrq.gov/

Screening

PHQ-9: http://www.pfizer.com/pfizer/phq-9/index.jsp

References

1. Karlin BE, Fuller JD. Meeting the mental health needs of older adults: implications for primary care practice. *Geriatrics*. 2007;62:26–35.

2. Frederick JT, Steinman LE, Prohaska T, et al. Community-based treatment of late life depression: an expert panel-informed literature review. *Am J Preventive Med*. 2007;33(3):222–249.

3. Lyness JM, Caine ER, King DA, Cox C, Yoediono Z. Psychiatric disorders in older primary care patients. *J Gen Intern Med*. 1999;14:249–254.

4. Frasure-Smith N, Lesperance F, Talajic M. Depression and 18-month prognosis after myocardial infarction. *Circulation*. 1995;91:999–1005.

5. Pennix BW, Beekman JE, Barrett J, et al. Depression and cardiac mortality: results from a community-based longitudinal study. *Arch Gen Psychiatry*. 2001;58:221–227.

6. Li C, Friedman B, Conwell Y. Validity of the Patient Health Questionnaire 2 (PHQ-2) in identifying major depression in older people. *J Am Geriatr Soc*. 2007;55:596–602.

7. Thibault JM, Steiner RWP. Efficient identification of adults with depression and dementia. *Am Fam Physician*. 2004;70:1101–1110.

8. Slaughter JR, Slaughter KA, Nichols D. Prevalence, clinical manifestations, etiology, and treatment of depression in Parkinson's disease. *J Neuropsychiatry Clin Neurosci*. 2001;13:187–196.

9. Emre M, Aarsland D, Brown R, et al. Clinical diagnostic criteria for dementia associated with Parkinson's disease. *Movement Disorders*. 2007;22(12):1689–1707.

10. Evans DL, Charney DS, Lewis L, et al. Mood disorders in the medically ill: scientific review and recommendations. *Biol Psychiatry*. 2005;58(3):175–189.

11. Lawhorne L, Ogle KS. Approaches to the office care of the older adults and the specter of dementia. *Prim Care Clin Office Pract.* 2005;32:599–618.

12. Bartels SJ, Drums AR, Oxman TE, et al. Evidence-based practices in geriatric mental health care: an overview of systematic reviews and meta-analyses. *Psychiatric Clin North Am.* 2003;26:971–990.

13. Reynolds CF III, Frank E, Perel JM. Nortriptyline and interpersonal psychotherapy as maintenance therapies for recurrent major depression: a randomized controlled trial in patients older than 59 years. *JAMA.* 1999;281(1):39–45.

14. Unützer J. Late-life depression. *N Engl J Med.* 2007;357:2269–2276.

15. Gum A, Arean PA, Hunkeler E, et al. Depression treatment preferences in older primary care patients. *Gerontologist.* 2006;46(1):14–22.

16. Unützer J, Katon W, Callahan CM, et al. Collaborative-care management of late-life depression in the primary care setting: a randomized controlled trial. *JAMA.* 2002;288:2836–2845.

17. Callahan CM, Kroenke K, Counsell SR, et al. Treatment of depression improves physical functioning in older adults. *J Am Geriatr Soc.* 2005;53(3):367–373.

18. Yaffe K. Treatment of neuropsychiatric symptoms in patients with dementia. *N Engl J Med.* 2007;357:1441–1443.

Chapter 18

The "difficult" patient

Yeshesvini Raman

Most physicians have encountered a number of "difficult" patients in their practices, in both inpatient and outpatient settings. Such patients often trigger different feelings in health care providers, such as frustration, agony, or annoyance. "Difficult" patients are some of the high utilizers of health care resources. A variety of factors can lead to a patient being categorized as "difficult," and few patients intend to be difficult: the interplay of patient, physician, staff, family, and circumstantial factors can all contribute. Several cases will be presented to illustrate this point.

The angry patient

Mr. J is always intimidating to the primary care secretary, Sally. He is typically loud and angry when coming in for his appointment. Sally goes out of her way to pay attention to the appointment schedule and tries hard to avoid encounters with him by taking her break accordingly. Mr. J speaks to his primary care physician in a loud, irate tone, and he rigorously questions each action and recommendation the physician makes. Staff members are usually glad when Mr. J leaves the office.

Patients with high hostility often cause negative feelings in health care providers, resulting in avoidant behaviors by staff and physicians. It is important to consider possible psychopathology that may underlie the patient's angry demeanor. Psychopathology commonly found in angry patients includes the following:[1]

- Bipolar disorders (irritable or manic type)
- Mild to moderate depressive disorder, especially among male patients
- Substance abuse (intoxication or withdrawal)
- Antisocial personality disorder
- Narcissistic personality disorder
- Post-traumatic stress disorder
- Traumatic brain injury

The demanding patient

Mr. P is a 56-year-old with chronic pain who calls the office at least twice a week demanding pain medications. Recently, he's been calling because he wants a wrist splint for self-diagnosed carpal tunnel syndrome. After he is prescribed the splint he is dissatisfied and calls back, stating that he has not received the correct splint. Out of frustration, the provider refers him to see an orthopedic surgeon.

Demanding patients question all treatment options presented by the provider and always seem more demanding than the typical patient with regard to health care. The demanding patient may complain or threaten legal and administrative action if his or her needs are not met. He or she may also repeatedly contact staff, demanding favors from them. Staff frustration heightens when such a patient appears.

Common causes or contributors to a patient's demanding demeanor include the following:

- Chronic pain
- Antisocial personality disorder
- Narcissistic personality disorder
- Underlying paranoia secondary to any of the following: schizophrenia, schizoaffective disorder, post-traumatic stress disorder, schizoid personality disorder, paranoid personality disorders
- Bipolar disorder
- Substance abuse or dependence

The noncompliant patient

Mrs. V is a 28-year-old woman with insulin-requiring type 2 diabetes. She weighs 342 lbs. She is admitted for non-ketotic acidosis for the third time in a year. Her blood sugar level is 1023, and her glycosylated hemoglobin is 16.2. She says she takes all her medications regularly, though her provider recalls that she never brings her glucometer in for her appointments. In the office, her fasting blood sugar readings have been in the 400s. Her family reports that Mrs. V eats large amounts of carbohydrate-rich food daily and does not take her insulin regularly.

Noncompliance can cause health professionals to feel belittled and incompetent. Causes of noncompliance could include the following:

- Mood disorders, commonly depressive disorders, passive suicidality, lack of motivation, poor energy level
- Psychotic disorder, paranoia regarding medications, ritualistic behavior and unusual beliefs, delusional thinking
- Learning disorder/mental retardation
- Psychosocial issues, including financial issues (e.g., inability to buy medications or follow a healthy diet)
- Factitious disorders—a conscious or unconscious need to be in an ongoing sick role

The "drama queen" (or king)

Dr. M starts seeing Ms. F regarding her new complaint of pain in the abdomen. When asked about any recent unusual diets, Ms. F starts to talk about her recent cruise to the Bahamas and how she met a new friend. She goes into lengthy details about all that she did on that cruise. Dr. M's multiple attempts to obtain more relevant details about her pain are ignored by Ms. F, who continues to describe her escapades in the Caribbean. With less than 5 minutes before her appointment ends, she starts to cry loudly about her pain and how it is affecting her. She also starts to writhe in pain, rolling around on the exam table. By the end of the appointment, Dr. M needs to call in extra staff to help calm Ms. F down.

Initial amusement and interest sparked by patients like Ms. F may turn to annoyance, causing physicians in continuity practice to start resenting and avoiding such patients. Because dramatic patients often go on and on talking about themselves in a grandiose fashion, or provide extensive and elaborate details in conversations, visits are often time-consuming and take the focus away from providing adequate care.

The differential diagnosis for dramatic patients should include the following:

- Mania or hypomania
- Histrionic personality disorder
- Narcissistic personality disorder
- Drug intoxication
- Somatization
- Psychotic symptoms
- Korsakoff's psychosis (e.g., confabulation)

The dissatisfied patient

Mr. A presents with a complaint of bilateral lower eyelid swelling. Dr. R diagnoses severe allergies and starts him on medication. Mr. A returns after 1 week with significantly less swelling, but he still reports that treatment has not helped: he wants a trial of a different medication. Dr. R reluctantly changes medications, but Mr. A returns a week later asking for a stronger medication. One week later the patient calls again with a request for a consultation with an expert allergist.

A few patients never seem to be content with the level or type of care the physician provides. These patients doubt the diagnosis, management, and alternatives and come with a long list of new or ongoing complaints that do not seem to improve with any treatment. Sometimes these patients start "doctor-shopping" to satisfy their needs. Physicians often feel overwhelmed by such patients and just want them to go away.

The differential diagnosis for the dissatisfied patient includes the following:

- Somatization disorder
- Body dysmorphic disorder
- Anxiety disorder
- Chronic pain
- Hypochondriasis

The needy patient

Mr. T, recently divorced, "drops in" every week requesting a refill of medications, wanting to discuss the side effects of medications, or needing ideas for diet and exercise to help control his hypertension. Despite home health visits to help with the healing of his foot ulcer, he has multiple questions for the primary care physician regarding the ongoing treatment of the ulcer.

The needy patient is often pleasant, causing the physician to feel a tremendous urge to help him or her. However, soon the patient may cause significant provider exhaustion as he or she seeks constant support and reassurance.

The differential diagnosis for needy patients includes the following:

- Somatization disorder
- Malingering
- Mood disorder
- Anxiety disorder
- Dependent personality disorder

The silent patient

Mr. P is a 65-year-old with a history of chronic obstructive pulmonary disease and alcohol dependence in remission of 4 years. Over the past year he has become very passive. His wife says that he usually keeps to himself; as she still is working, she is not able to give much information about how Mr. P spends his day. Vital signs are all normal, except blood pressure, which is 150/86. All of his answers are monosyllabic.

Initial empathy from the provider may be replaced by shorter and shorter visit times, as it is very hard and time-consuming to elicit history from a silent patient. Most of the history is then obtained from family, which can also be very limited in detail.

The differential diagnosis to consider for silent patients includes the following:

- Dementia
- Pseudodementia (e.g., from major depressive disorder)
- Polypharmacy (e.g., sedating medications)

- Medical etiology (e.g., CVA, Parkinson's disease, cognitive disorder, hearing loss)
- Anxiety disorder
- Post-traumatic stress disorder
- Social anxiety disorder
- Hypochondriasis
- Fear of getting sick or worsening of symptoms
- Cultural and language barriers

The seductive patient

Ms. M is a 43-year-old single woman who, during her exam, comments on what a good-looking doctor Dr. Y is. She continues to say that she has not had an intimate relationship in a few years and how she has always longed to be with somebody like Dr. Y.

Suggestive and sexually inappropriate behaviors of a patient can lead to changes in a provider's attitudes and approaches, such as being overly involved or, conversely, avoidant. The physician–patient boundaries may be blurred. Unwanted referrals to subspecialty may also be made to decrease the burden of patient interactions. At times, providers may give in to requests for medications to avoid conflict.

Seductive behaviors may be seen in patients with the following:

- Bipolar disorder hypomania/mania
- Post-traumatic stress disorder
- Borderline personality disorder
- Histrionic personality disorder

Approaches to the management of difficult patients

There is almost no patient who aspires to be "difficult." Patients who present with the above-described inappropriate behaviors generally do so because their needs are unmet or have not been met to their satisfaction. On the other hand, with the complexity of the psychopathological characters these patients may possess, management of these patients is often beyond the excellent capacity of an individual physician. The following points are suggestions to enhance effective interactions with those patients (refer also to Chapter 1, "Communicating Effectively with Patients"):

- Schedule longer visits to understand issues better.
- Involve family members/social workers.
- Consider a multidisciplinary approach to management—for example, in a patient with diabetes, involve nursing, nutrition, endocrine teams, and podiatry as appropriate.

- Ask open-ended questions to get the most history.
- Set clear limits for demanding, seductive, and angry patients, and do not deviate from the limits that have been set. Consider establishing a contract for ongoing treatment, outlining expectations of appropriate patient and provider behavior.
- Clarify patient symptoms, expectations, and treatment goals and plans.
- Reinforce positive behaviors.
- Maintain communication among providers to limit splitting. Avoid gossiping about patients or their problems with other staff members.
- Refer patients for evaluation to diagnose treatable Axis I or Axis II psychiatry issues. Some patients may get upset or offended that a psychiatrist has been consulted. Before planning consults, discuss with the patient why and to whom he or she is being referred—for example, talk about the referral as a way to get a different perspective on issues, or to get help for what emotional issues or problems may arise. (Refer to Chapter 2, "When to Call for Psychiatric Help.")
- Consider a trial of medications to help with treatment of depression, bipolar disorder, anxiety disorder, and so forth. (Refer to Chapter 4, "Overview of Psychopharmacologic Therapies.")
- Screen for substance use disorders, and refer the patient to a substance abuse clinic if any are identified.
- Establish a positive alliance with the patient; work as a team in partnership to help resolve issues.
- Acknowledge difficulties with diagnosis and treatment.

Despite all efforts and with the best physician intent, some patients may remain difficult to work with. If reasonable effort has been made, when patients and providers remain frustrated and at odds with one another, seeking a second opinion, referring to subspecialty, or even referring to another primary provider may be the best option to maintain a healthy therapeutic alliance in achieving overall treatment goals.

Encounters with difficult patients can be extremely challenging and exhausting to staff and providers. A patient perceived as "difficult" in any setting poses significant issues and can interfere with optimal care. The provider's ability to recognize these patterns of behavior early, provide appropriate interventions, and avoid becoming angry or unnecessarily frustrated can help. Ideally, these patients can be managed without elaborate interventions.

Reference

1. *Diagnostic and Statistical Manual of Mental Disorders, Fourth Edition, Text Revision* (DSM-IV-TR). Washington, DC: American Psychiatric Association; 2000.

Chapter 19

The patient with an unusual presentation

Jane P. Gagliardi and Wei Jiang

Sometimes patients present with symptoms that persist, symptoms that do not fit neatly into a diagnostic category, or syndromes that stump the physician. Patients may produce symptoms or even seem to defy the physician's best efforts to promote health. This chapter will discuss two types of unusual presentations: factitious disorders and catatonia.

Clinical scenario 1

Ms. W, a 42-year-old woman, presents to the emergency department with fevers and nausea. She has had multiple emergency department visits and hospitalizations with skin infections and abscesses, including mixed Gram-negative and methicillin-resistant Staphylococcus aureus (MRSA) infections that have required home IV antibiotic therapy, for which she has had a central venous port placed. She has a history of chronic pain, for which she takes opiate pain medications, and depressive disorder; both of these issues are managed by her psychiatrist.

Ms. W is a well-developed, well-nourished woman who is in no acute distress, but she is febrile to 40°C and has multiple areas of induration and erythema consistent with cellulitis and abscesses scattered over her chest, abdomen, thighs, and left arm. Inspection of the central venous port site reveals erythema and some purulent material. Blood cultures are drawn, she is started on vancomycin and piperacillin/tazobactam, and she is admitted to Dr. C's service for further evaluation and management. During the first two hospital days, despite broad-spectrum antibiotic therapy, Ms. W continues to spike high fevers. Blood cultures return positive for mixed Gram-positive cocci and Gram-negative rods, and Dr. C is concerned about the possibility of central line infection. He shares this concern with Ms. W, but she refuses to have the central venous port removed.

Dr. C orders a transesophageal echocardiogram, which is negative for evidence of valvular vegetations or abscesses. Dr. C becomes suspicious that Ms. W may be manipulating her line or otherwise causing her own infection and requests a room search and a 24-hour sitter for observation and monitoring, given the grave consequences of intravascular infection and sepsis. Ms. W defervesces, and Dr. C keeps her in the hospital to complete her course of antibiotics.

Factitious disorder: Background

Providing care to patients with suspected factitious disorders requires an open mind, careful scrutiny of other possible etiologies, and hard work to align with the patient when possible. Though sometimes secondary gain may be apparent, in many cases it is not possible to know the patient's underlying motives. In most cases, minimizing harm and optimizing rapport are the most realistic goals of treatment.

Patients with factitious disorder may present with any number of medical or psychological conditions. "Professional patients" may provide excellent histories that can deceive the most experienced clinician[1] and may withhold information, such as past medical records or visits to multiple other providers, that would lead to the correct diagnosis.

The keys to diagnosing factitious disorders are awareness and evidence-gathering. Gathering evidence is often exhausting and is best achieved through repeated and detailed reviews of systems, social histories, and (with patient permission) collection of previous medical records and contact with other clinicians and pharmacies. While acknowledging the patient's right to privacy and confidentiality, ethical and legal counsel may be necessary for consideration of room searches when significant morbidity or mortality is imminent.[2]

Factitious symptoms and signs may co-exist with true physical (or psychological) symptoms and signs; thus, the diagnosis of factitious disorder should always be made after reasonable exclusion of true medical conditions and/or true mental disorders, and the clinician should remain alert to the possibility of new or additional medical problems that may arise.

Factitious disorder: Differential diagnosis

The importance of ruling out actual medical diseases or conditions cannot be overstated, even in a patient who is known to have factitious disorder and presents routinely in a similar fashion.

Factitious disorder and malingering are both disorders in which patients create, or make up, signs and symptoms. In malingering, symptoms are produced for an obvious external incentive (e.g., to get out of jail, to avoid military service, to obtain disability, for the purposes of litigation); patients frequently stop self-inflicting signs and symptoms when the risk of illness becomes too great. On the other hand, patients with factitious disorder have no obvious external incentive apart from assuming or maintaining the sick role[3] and can present with serious and complex medical problems.

Malingering and factitious disorder differ from somatoform disorders by the voluntary production of signs and symptoms. Patients with somatoform disorders (e.g., conversion disorder) do not intentionally produce their symptoms; there is no obvious secondary gain, and symptoms usually have a direct temporal relation or symbolic reference to specific emotional conflict.

Features that may lead to detection of factitious disorder

Certain common characteristics among patients with factitious disorders include the following:

- Presentations that do not conform to one identifiable medical condition or mental disorder
- Indifference (i.e., patients are not bothered by the severity of their presentations)
- Multiple admissions or repeated presentations to emergency departments, often across states (this can be difficult to elicit, as patients may not cooperate with efforts to seek medical records)
- Disruptive behavior
- Reluctance to meet with psychiatry consultant
- Few visitors despite prolonged hospitalizations
- History or present employment in a medical field
- Medical sophistication
- Experience with a serious illness in adolescence or childhood
- History of multiple surgeries (with identifiable scars) often complicated by infectious diseases or poor healing
- Fake and multiple identities
- Reluctance to allow collection of past medical records
- Pattern of discharge against medical advice

Factitious disorder: Management

Always be vigilant for the development of complications with potential mortality and morbidity. On the other hand, it is important to avoid ordering potentially harmful diagnostic tests or treatments in the absence of clear evidence of disease. Getting at the underlying root of the factitious disorder may never be possible, but when the physician suspects factitious disorder, it is important to implement practices that will help the patient to stay safe, such as 24-hour observation with a sitter and room searches for safety.

Factitious disorder: Common pitfalls

Maintaining an open and nonjudgmental attitude can be helpful in the management of patients with factitious disorder. Many times when a patient realizes the physician suspects factitious disorder, he or she requests discharge against medical advice (AMA); it is therefore important to accomplish necessary treatments before informing patients of suspicion. If the patient requests discharge AMA, it is a good idea to obtain psychiatric consultation to rule out the presence of suicidal or homicidal ideation. Petition via legal procedure may be needed if the patient has an imminent life-threatening condition. In other instances, psychiatric consultation may be helpful to elucidate underlying issues or etiologies.

Clinical scenario 2

The inpatient cardiology service requests a consult from the combined medicine and psychiatry service for Ms. C, a 45-year-old woman with a 15-year history of idiopathic cardiomyopathy, ejection fraction 15%, who also carries a diagnosis of depressive disorder. She was admitted to the hospital from a nursing home with exacerbation of heart failure. Shortly after admission, Ms. C became mute and minimally responsive, refusing to eat.

On examination, Ms. C opens her eyes spontaneously at times but will not answer questions, nor will she initiate a conversation. She resists the examiner's efforts to open her eyes. She demonstrates waxy flexibility (arms remain elevated for a while after the examiner lifts them). Her outpatient doctor and family members note that Ms. C has had a couple of similar episodes over the past year. A trial of scheduled lorazepam is initiated and results in reduced muteness, negativism, and immobility, as well as improved oral intake.

Catatonia: Background

Catatonia is one of the most perplexing of psychiatric syndromes and may present a difficult diagnostic dilemma. It is described as follows: "For no apparent reason, a person may become mute, freeze for minutes or hours on end without any discernable awareness of the outside world, appear seemingly impervious to pain, and allow their limbs to be bent in all sorts of awkward positions."[4]

Catatonia is associated with a large and heterogeneous group of conditions. Many psychiatric problems may result in catatonia, including schizophrenia, depression, conversion, acute stress disorder, or even hysteria. The list of physical problems associated with catatonia is also substantial,[5,6] and new associations continue to be reported, including neurological disorders involving focal lesions of the brain stem, basal ganglia, thalamus, limbic system, and temporal and frontal lobes due to encephalitis, tumor, hemorrhagic or ischemic stoke, and other vascular lesions, and diffuse cerebral disorders due to closed head injury, encephalomalacia, epilepsy, and neurosyphilis. Catatonia has also been associated with systemic disorders including hormonal disorders; vitamin deficiency; porphyria; systemic lupus erythematosus; infection; liver, renal, or heart failure; carbon monoxide poisoning; drugs of abuse or intoxication; neuroleptic medications; and benzodiazepine withdrawal. Disulfiram and cyclosporine toxicity have been associated with catatonia. Perplexingly, in one series 40% of patients with catatonia had no identifiable psychiatric or organic causes.[7]

While catatonia was once thought to be a cerebral manifestation of extrapyramidal motor disorder, catatonia is currently understood as a disruption in the circuit among the orbitofrontal lobe, especially on the right side; the limbic system; the amygdala; the hypothalamus; the basal ganglia; and the vagus nerve. The disruption is thought to be caused by extremely intense fear, organic injury of any component of the loop, or both.[4,8]

Prevalence and prognosis of catatonia

The prevalence of catatonia is poorly defined due to a lack of systematic studies and poor recognition. One study suggests that 9% of patients admitted to an adult psychiatric unit presented with catatonia, and two-thirds of those cases were associated with medical conditions.[6] Another study of patients admitted to a neurology ward with catatonia over 12 years found that 20% of those catatonic syndromes were due to general medical conditions.[7]

It is believed that catatonia represents an increased severity of diseases in general.[8] Failure to institute treatment early in the course of the condition is associated with a poor prognosis. The most severe form of catatonia can be fatal, especially if treatment is not prompt and effective. Studies of catatonia have reported recovery rates ranging from 12% to more than 40% regardless of the treatment administered; death may result from associated medical conditions (e.g., malnutrition, pulmonary embolism, infection).[9]

Catatonia: Differential diagnosis

Symptoms

The diagnosis of catatonia is not difficult for a vigilant clinician. Catatonia is characterized by the presence of a variety of behavioral and motor traits, occurring acutely or subacutely with fluctuation of symptoms. There are two forms of catatonia. Stuporous catatonia, by far the more common form, is characterized by immobility, mutism, and many other symptoms, such as negativism (opposition to suggestion or advice; behavior opposite to that appropriate to a specific situation), echopraxia (spasmodic and involuntary imitation of the movements of others), echolalia (automatic repetition of what is said), waxy flexibility, and withdrawal. Stuporous catatonia is represented in the vignette at the beginning of this section. Excited catatonia, by contrast, is characterized by a bizarre, purposeless, and frenzied hyperactivity; it may be associated with impulsivity, combativeness, and autonomic instability.[10]

Diagnosis

The diagnosis of catatonia due to a general medical condition requires the presence of a potentially explanatory medical condition along with the following symptoms: immobility or restlessness, unusual movements (such as waxy flexibility, considered a hallmark of catatonia), mutism, or unusual speech patterns.[3]

It is important to consider catatonia when a patient is apparently awake but unresponsive to external stimuli. It is also imperative to consider possible medical causes for catatonia, even when there is a known psychiatric condition.

Patients with catatonia are often unable to provide a history. For this reason, it is important to seek information from collateral sources. Family members can confirm the presence of typical primary features of stuporous catatonia but may not always be able to recognize excited episodes, which may be short-lived and may precipitate collapse with exhaustion.

Differential

It is important to distinguish stuporous catatonia from akinetic mutism and from stupor of other causes, particularly medical or neurological causes. Patients with akinetic mutism will be immobile and mute but will not demonstrate waxy flexibility, negativism, or other symptoms typical of catatonia. Stupor due to noncatatonic causes is readily distinguished from catatonia by level of alertness: stuporous catatonia patients remain alert, whereas otherwise stuporous patients are somnolent.

It is possible to distinguish excited catatonia from mania by paying attention to purposeful activity and involvement with others: patients with excited catatonia remain isolative and uninvolved with others, whereas patients with excited mania continue to affiliate with others.

In an emergency setting, consider common treatable causes of catatonia, including neuroleptic malignant syndrome (NMS), encephalitis, nonconvulsive status epilepticus, and acute psychosis.

Catatonia: Management

Treatment of catatonia is directed at the underlying cause, which can be identified only with a thorough medical evaluation. Should emergent treatment be required, lorazepam (2 mg dose) or another benzodiazepine in equivalent dosing given parenterally is generally effective. Some physicians use a "test dose" of lorazepam to demonstrate the diagnosis of catatonia—catatonic patients will appear to activate or "wake up" with such administration. In cases of life-threatening catatonia, electroconvulsive therapy (ECT) may be used.

Catatonia: Common pitfalls

- Because NMS may occur in patients with symptoms and signs of catatonia, use of neuroleptics should be avoided if possible unless the etiology is clearly a primary psychotic disorder.
- Generally, the onset of catatonia merits hospitalization, on an involuntary basis if necessary, for the diagnostic workup and initiation of treatment.

Useful resources

Asher R. Munchausen's syndrome. *Lancet.* 1951;1:339–341.

Pollock RCG. Investigation of chronic diarrhoea [comment]. *Gut.* 2004;53:770.

Shelton JH, Santa Ana CA, Thompson DR, Emmet M, Fordtran JS. Factitious diarrhea induced by stimulant laxatives: accuracy of diagnosis by clinical reference thin layer chromatography. *Clin Chem.* 2007;53(1):85–90.

Wallach J. Laboratory diagnosis of factitious disorders. *Arch Intern Med.* 1994;154:1690–1696.

References

1. Sadock BJ, Sadock VA. *Kaplan & Sadock's Synopsis of Psychiatry* (9th ed). Philadelphia: Lippincott Williams & Wilkins; 2003:670.

2. Folks DG, Freeman AM. Munchausen's syndrome and other factitious illness. Psychiatr *Clin North Am.* 1985;8(2):263–278.

3. *Diagnostic and Statistical Manual of Mental Disorders, Fourth Edition, Text Revision* (DSM-IV-TR). Washington, DC: American Psychiatric Association; 2000.

4. Moskowitz AK. "Scared stiff": catatonia as an evolutionary-based fear response. *Psychol Rev.* 2004;111(4):984–1002.

5. Carroll BT, Anfinson TJ, Kennedy JC, Yendrek R, Boutros M, Bilon A. Catatonic disorder due to general medical conditions. *J Neuropsychiatry Clin Neurosci.* 1994;6:122–133.

6. Rosebush PI, Hildebrand AM, Furlong BG, Mazurek MF. Catatonic syndrome in a general psychiatric inpatient population: frequency, clinical presentation, and response to lorazepam. *J Clin Psychiatry.* 1990;51(9):357–362.

7. Barnes MP, Saunders M, Walls TJ, Saunders I, Kirk CA. The syndrome of Karl Ludwig Kahlbaum. *J Neurol Neurosurg Psychiatry.* 1986;49:991–996.

8. Rogers D. Catatonia: a contemporary approach. *J Neuropsychiatry Clin Neurosci.* 1991;3:334–340.

9. Manu P, Suarez RE, Barnett BJ. *Handbook of Medicine in Psychiatry.* Washington, DC: American Psychiatry Publishing Inc.; 2006:142–143.

10. Carroll BT. Kahlbaum's catatonia revisited. *Psychiatry Clin Neurosci.* 2001;55(5):431–436.

Chapter 20

The patient who refuses treatment

Sarah K. Rivelli

Clinical scenario

Mr. O, a 78-year-old widower with coronary artery disease, hypertension, hyperlipidemia, diabetes, and prostate cancer, requests an urgent appointment with Dr. R for fatigue and shortness of breath walking up the stairs to his front door and to the mailbox, which is new for him. He "forgot" his last two scheduled appointments, which he missed. On exam his pulse is irregularly irregular and he has crackles at the lung bases and edema to his shins. An ECG shows atrial fibrillation. Dr. R tells Mr. O he has an abnormal heart rhythm and a provisional diagnosis of heart failure and recommends inpatient admission for evaluation. The patient states, "I've been hospitalized enough. I just want to go home."

Background

The right to refuse treatment is an exercise of basic constitutional rights, especially the right to self-determination. The assessment of a patient who refuses treatment is complex and requires evaluation of the patient's preferences and values as well as medical decision-making capacity. The physician is bound by competing principles: the duty to help the patient and the duty to protect his or her autonomy, one of the guiding ethical principles in American medicine.

Refusal of treatment is more often due to a failure in communication than a lack of capacity.[1] It is therefore important to work to repair communication, establish trust, and negotiate with the patient. Primary care providers generally get to know their patients over time and have established trust; thus, they can participate in discussions with specialty consultants and advocate for their patients.

If a patient is found to lack capacity, a substitute decision-maker must be sought. If advance directives are present, turning to the named surrogate decision-maker or following the instructions in the directives is warranted. It is important to be aware of state laws, as some states recognize only legally appointed health care proxies as surrogate decision-makers, whereas others allow family members to step in as decision-makers.

Conducting an appropriate capacity assessment

Approach to history-taking

Physicians are bound by law and medical ethics to obtain informed consent from patients before commencing treatment. Decision-making capacity for consent to treatment requires that patients do the following[2]:

- Communicate a choice
- Understand the relevant information
- Appreciate the medical consequences of the situation
- Be able to reason about treatment choices

Therefore, the physician assessing capacity must have a clear understanding of the proposed treatment, risks, benefits, and possible outcomes before conducting the capacity assessment.

In communicating a choice, the patient must be able to clearly indicate a preference. A patient with an inability to communicate a clear choice due to ambivalence or vacillation would lack capacity for that decision. Patients have the right to make "unreasonable" choices, however, as long as they are able to demonstrate understanding of their current health condition, the recommended treatment and its benefits and risks, alternative treatments, and consequences of nontreatment. The patient must acknowledge the medical condition and the likely consequences or outcomes. An individual who lacks insight or denies the existence of illness cannot make valid treatment decisions regarding that illness.

Repeat evaluation at different times may be helpful. Collateral information from family members or close acquaintances is necessary; the family may also help the patient understand the proposed treatment and alternatives.

In assessing capacity, the risk–benefit ratio of the suggested intervention is important. If a patient refuses a low-risk/high-benefit intervention, close scrutiny of his or her understanding is called for. For example, if Mr. O refuses a transthoracic echocardiogram (a low-risk procedure) recommended for assessment of treatable heart failure (possibly high benefit in terms of symptoms and mortality), his decision-making capacity bears scrutiny. Any high-risk procedure (e.g., cardioversion, surgery, or another invasive procedure) requires close scrutiny of the patient's understanding, regardless of his or her willingness to consent.

Competence versus capacity

Incompetence is a verdict rendered in a court of law and can lead to the appointment of a guardian to make decisions regarding the individual's "person" and even property. Physicians are not able to make decisions regarding competence but are able to perform evaluations of capacity, the scope of which is limited to the medical decision at hand. If a patient is found to lack capacity, consent must be obtained from a proxy decision-maker. A health care proxy or durable power of attorney named in an advance directive is invoked when a patient is deemed to lack decision-making capacity. In the absence of an advance directive of health care proxy, a substitute decision-maker may be a family member. Some state statutes specify a hierarchy in which family members may become substitute decision-makers; generally the order is spouse, adult children, parents, siblings, and then other relatives. The goal in these cases is to honor the patient's autonomy, ideally with proxies or relatives who keep the patient's preferences in mind when making medical decisions.

Psychiatric disorders

Psychiatric assessment is not generally required as part of a capacity assessment, as the presence of psychiatric illness does not necessarily lead to a lack of decisional capacity. However, if mental illness is known or suspected, psychiatric evaluation may help determine whether the illness affects the patient's medical decision-making capacity. Not surprisingly, moderate to severe cognitive impairment is associated with lack of capacity. In fact, an MMSE score of less than 19/30 is highly likely to be associated with lack of capacity.[3]

Patients with active psychiatric disorders often lack insight into their psychiatric condition and may not believe that they have a mental illness or need treatment. This unique situation is handled independently from capacity for nonpsychiatric medical decision-making. Under involuntary detention or civil commitment laws, which vary state by state, individuals with mental illness may be detained against their wishes in cases of imminent danger to themselves or others and/or inability to provide for their own basic needs. The provider may seek involuntary psychiatric hospitalization for a patient meeting established criteria, and the decision to "hold" the patient is made by the court. **Civil commitment applies only to psychiatric evaluation and treatment and does not allow for medical treatment without consent.** If a patient lacks capacity for medical decision-making, a surrogate decision-maker must still be sought for the medical intervention in question, regardless of involuntary commitment for psychiatric treatment. For instance, imagine a patient with schizophrenia who is involuntarily committed for psychiatric treatment also has a non-healing diabetic foot ulcer. When an amputation is recommended by the surgical consultant, consent by either the patient (if he or she is deemed to have capacity to consent to the procedure) or by a surrogate decision-maker (if the patient lacks capacity to consent) is necessary for the amputation to be performed.

Differential diagnosis

A patient may refuse treatment due to lack of understanding, misconceptions, or lack of trust. The patient may simply be making a reasonable decision in line with his or her values and goals, though his or her preferences may be unusual or uncommon. If a patient is found to lack decision-making capacity, potential causes should be examined, including the following:

- A treatable and reversible cognitive impairment (such as delirium)
- A progressive or permanent cognitive impairment (such as dementia)
- A treatable psychiatric disorder (such as depression, mania, or psychosis)
- Severe personality disorders resulting in impaired judgment

Thorough evaluation of the nature and extent of cognitive or psychiatric deficits may illuminate the patient's need for a permanent surrogate decision-maker, such as a guardian, if there is no proxy named in a legal document such as an advance directive.

Intervention strategies

After taking time to discuss in lay language the indications, risks, and benefits of the procedure proposed, the provider must elicit the patient's understanding of his or her condition and the various options for treatment (or not). Empathy, respect, and a strong physician–patient relationship may serve to overcome the conflict without the need for a formal capacity evaluation. There may be an opportunity to negotiate with the patient—for example, by focusing on treating pain or anxiety prior to sending the patient for an invasive procedure.[1] Patients with cognitive deficits may benefit from careful efforts at education, including providing information in verbal and written forms.

Emergency situations

The right to refuse treatment and the requirement for informed consent are usually waived in medical or surgical emergencies. A provider acting in good faith to save life or prevent imminent serious harm in an emergency, when it is impossible to obtain consent from the patient or to identify an appropriate proxy, is generally not liable for failure to obtain informed consent. However, if the patient has previously made his or her preferences known, such as via DNR/DNI status or a request for no blood transfusions, such preferences should be honored.

Common pitfalls

- The most common error in approaching a patient who refuses care is to move directly to a capacity assessment.[1] Efforts to improve communication, build trust, and provide adequate education may replace the need to evaluate capacity. If a lack of capacity is suspected, communication remains essential to help the patient assent and cooperate with treatment, even if consent is granted by a surrogate decision-maker.

- Providers frequently confuse the terms *competence*, which is a legal determination, and *capacity*, which is a clinical determination and generally more limited in scope pertaining to the intervention or treatment proposed.
- Providers should not assume that a patient lacks capacity simply because of mental illness. However, cognitive deficits and dementia and their negative impact on decision-making capacity are generally underestimated.[3]
- Lack of capacity may be temporary or limited in scope; thus, repeat evaluation is often necessary.

References

1. Simon JR. Refusal of care: the physician-patient relationship and decisionmaking capacity. *Ann Emerg Med.* 2007;50:456–461.
2. Appelbaum PS. Assessment of patients' competence to consent to treatment. *N Engl J Med.* 2007;357:1834–1840.
3. Raymont V, Bingley W, Buchanan A, et al. Prevalence of mental incapacity in medical inpatients and associated risk factors: cross-sectional study. *Lancet.* 2004;364:1421–1427.

Chapter 21

Overview of the practice of psychotherapy

Moria J. Smoski and Thomas R. Lynch

Psychotherapy, or "talk therapy," is an important tool in the arsenal of treatments for mental disorders or enhancement of coping skills for people in general. Dating back to Freud, talk therapies have been used to reduce psychological symptoms and to promote improved functioning and well-being. A number of psychotherapeutic modalities have been developed over the past century. Several have been found to be as effective or more effective than medications for certain disorders. Though every case differs, there are several good reasons to consider referring a medical patient for psychotherapy in lieu of, or in addition to, prescribing medications:

1. Psychotherapy can be an effective option for treating psychological conditions when medication interactions are a concern or side effects are not well tolerated.
2. Psychotherapy allows a patient to address the broader psychosocial impact of a comorbid medical condition.
3. Psychotherapy has been shown to be the most appropriate first-line treatment for some disorders (e.g., personality disorders).

Psychotherapies can be broadly divided into treatments that target a patient's *thoughts*, *behaviors*, or *manners of relating*. These treatment targets correspond to cognitive, behavioral, and psychoanalytic or supportive therapies, respectively. Though successful treatments undoubtedly affect all three targets, many treatments draw their primary theoretical basis from one or two of these targets.

Cognitive therapies

Cognitive therapies are based on the theoretical model that a person's thoughts and beliefs invoke an emotional response, which in turn evokes a behavioral response or action tendency. From this perspective, psychopathology develops from thoughts or beliefs that are chronically maladaptive or distorted. For example, a person who habitually engages in catastrophic thinking (e.g., "This situation is awful! I'll never get over it!") may find himself or herself feeling chronically anxious or sad. Cognitive therapy focuses on recognizing, testing, and modifying these thoughts to cause emotional and behavioral change.

Cognitive therapy has been applied to a wide variety of clinical populations and diagnoses and is one of the best-studied psychotherapies at present. Cognitive therapy has shown at least equal effectiveness to pharmacotherapy in the treatment of depression,[1] generalized anxiety disorder,[2] panic disorder,[3] and obsessive-compulsive disorder,[4] among others. Cognitive therapy has also been shown effective in reducing the symptoms of several pain-related medical conditions, including chronic pain,[5] fibromyalgia,[6] and temporomandibular disorders.[7] However, data increasingly suggest that the salient mechanism of change in cognitive therapy relates to the development of metacognition (i.e., responding to negative thoughts as transitory events rather than as inherent aspects of self or as necessarily true) rather than change in the dysfunctional attitude per se.[8] Based on these observations, newer variants of cognitive therapy include mindfulness-based cognitive therapy (MBCT) and acceptance and commitment therapy, each adding a focus on metacognition. These interventions show tremendous promise in extending the effectiveness of cognitive therapy and reducing relapse in affected populations. In short, a referral for cognitive therapy is appropriate for a wide range of affective and pain-related conditions.

Behavioral therapies

Behavioral therapies use the principles of classical and operant conditioning to modify problematic behaviors and habits. Therapists help patients to establish environmental conditions and consequences that can shape voluntary behavior (operant conditioning) and to change behaviors based on antecedent conditions (classical conditioning). One example of a successful behavioral approach is exposure treatments for anxiety. Guided by the therapist, patients are gradually exposed to a feared stimulus (e.g., images of spiders for arachnophobia; a dirty stairwell banister for obsessive-compulsive disorder with contamination fears) but encouraged to forego any typical but problematic responses (e.g., flight, excessive hand washing), allowing the anxiety to subside over time. With repeated exposure in the absence of safety behaviors, the conditioned connection between the stimulus and the anxious emotional response begins to extinguish and new associations are developed. This therapeutic approach is highly effective for anxiety disorders, including obsessive-compulsive disorder[9] and post-traumatic stress disorder.[10] Given the effectiveness of even single-session treatments of specific phobias,[11] a referral for behavioral therapy is quite appropriate for patients who, for example, have blood-injection phobias that interfere with medical treatment.

Cognitive-behavioral therapy

Cognitive and behavioral approaches are often combined in a single treatment package (e.g., cognitive-behavioral therapy). However, recent component analysis research suggests that behavioral activation and automatic thought modification are equally effective; both components used together are no more effective in preventing relapse than when used alone.[12] Specific combinations of cognitive and behavioral techniques have been developed to target specific conditions. For example, dialectical behavior therapy[13] incorporates both acceptance-based (e.g., mindfulness) and change-oriented (e.g., behavioral exposure) techniques to reduce ineffective action tendencies linked with dysregulated emotions and has been shown to successfully target self-injury and suicide attempts among individuals with borderline personality disorder.[14,15]

Psychoanalytic therapy

Psychoanalytic treatments focus on the dynamics of unconscious intrapersonal processes that can evoke anxious or depressive symptoms and interfere with interpersonal relationships. Several short-term therapies based on psychodynamic principles have been developed in the past several decades that have shown effectiveness in treating a variety of disorders. In clinical trials, interpersonal psychotherapy has been effective in treating depression[16] and bulimia nervosa,[17] and mentalization-based treatment has shown effectiveness for treating personality disorders.[18] Brief psychodynamic therapy[19] uses the dynamic principles of transference as well as an active therapeutic alliance to correct interpersonal problems in other aspects of the patient's life.

Psychoanalytic treatments have traditionally lagged behind cognitive and behavioral treatments in the number of empirical tests of their efficacy, but more treatments will likely demonstrate efficacy as the literature grows.

Supportive therapy

Supportive therapies focus on providing elements common across many psychological treatments, including building a positive "working alliance" or therapeutic relationship between patient and therapist, facilitating the expression of emotion, and offering encouragement in coping with current stressors. Given its grounding in common principles across treatments, supportive therapy can be applied to many different kinds of patients and can be employed as a general strategy by even nonpsychiatric providers. However, it may lack techniques to target specific conditions.

Brief therapy

In addition to the treatments above, several brief therapies (e.g., one to six sessions) can be effective for focusing on specific problem situations or to enhance other treatments. *Solution-focused brief therapy* foregoes a focus on the causes and contributors of problems in favor of generating specific pathways out of difficult situations. Solution-focused therapy has been applied to populations ranging from depressed college students to recidivistic prisoners, with generally positive, if not conclusive, empirical support.[20] *Motivational interviewing*[21] is a technique of eliciting change in problematic behaviors (e.g., substance use, overeating) such that change is driven more by the patient's inherent motivation and less by pressure or direction of the therapist or provider. It can be used as a stand-alone treatment or as a means of preparing patients for more extensive intervention and is a technique that the nonpsychiatric provider can learn to employ in everyday practice.

Summary

Numerous effective psychotherapeutic interventions are available for treatment of psychiatric difficulties in patients with and without comorbid medical conditions. Referrals for psychotherapy are appropriate whenever emotional, behavioral, or other psychiatric symptoms interfere with a patient's medical care, level of functioning, or quality of life.

Acknowledgment

M. J. Smoski's work on this chapter was partially funded through T32 MH070448.

References

1. Hollon SD, DeRubeis RJ, Evans MD, et al. Cognitive therapy and pharmacotherapy for depression: singly and in combination. *Arch Gen Psychiatry.* 1992;49:774–781.

2. Mitte K. Meta-analysis of cognitive-behavioral treatments for generalized anxiety disorder: a comparison with pharmacotherapy. *Psychol Bull.* 2005;131:785–795.

3. Mitte K. A meta-analysis of the efficacy of psycho- and pharmacotherapy in panic disorder with and without agoraphobia. *J Affect Disorders.* 2005;88:27–45.

4. Sousa MB, Isolan LR, Oliveira RR, Manfro GG, Cordioli AV. A randomized clinical trial of cognitive-behavioral group therapy and sertraline in the treatment of obsessive-compulsive disorder. *J Clin Psychiatry.* 2006;67:1133–1139.

5. Hoffman BM, Papas RK, Chatkoff DK, Kerns RD. Meta-analysis of psychological interventions for chronic low back pain. *Health Psychol.* 2007;26:1–9.

6. Thieme K, Flor H, Turk DC. Psychological pain treatment in fibromyalgia syndrome: efficacy of operant behavioural and cognitive behavioural treatments. *Arthritis Res Therapy.* 2006;8:R121.

7. Turner JA, Mancl L, Aaron LA. Short- and long-term efficacy of brief cognitive-behavioral therapy for patients with chronic temporomandibular disorder pain: a randomized, controlled trial. *Pain.* 2006;121:181–194.

8. Teasdale JD, Moore RG, Hayhurst H, Pope M, Williams S, Segal ZV. Metacognitive awareness and prevention of relapse in depression: empirical evidence. *J Consult Clin Psych.* 2002;70:275–287.

9. Foa EB, Liebowitz MR, Kozak MJ, et al. Randomized, placebo-controlled trial of exposure and ritual prevention, clomipramine, and their combination

in the treatment of obsessive-compulsive disorder. *Am J Psychiatry.* 2005;162:151–161.

10. Rothbaum BO, Schwartz AC. Exposure therapy for posttraumatic stress disorder. *Am J Psychother.* 2002;56:59–75.

11. Öst L-G, Hellström K, Kaver A. One versus five sessions of exposure in the treatment of injection phobia. *Behav Ther.* 1992;23:263–282.

12. Dimidjian S, Hollon SD, Dobson KS, et al. Randomized trial of behavioral activation, cognitive therapy, and antidepressant medication in the acute treatment of adults with major depression. *J Consult Clin Psych.* 2006;74:658–670.

13. Linehan MM. *Cognitive-Behavioral Treatment of Borderline Personality Disorder.* New York: Guilford Press; 1993.

14. Linehan MM, Comtois KA, Murray AM, et al. Two-year randomized controlled trial and follow-up of dialectical behavior therapy vs therapy by experts for suicidal behaviors and borderline personality disorder. *Arch Gen Psychiatry.* 2006;63:757–766.

15. Lynch TR, Trost WT, Salsman N, Linehan MM. Dialectical behavior therapy for borderline personality disorder. *Ann Rev Clin Psychol.* 2007;3:181–205.

16. Elkin I, Shea MT, Watkins JT, et al. National Institute of Mental Health Treatment of Depression Collaborative Research Program. General effectiveness of treatments. *Arch Gen Psychiatry.* 1989;46:971–983.

17. Fairburn CG, Jones R, Peveler RC, Hope RA, O'Connor M. Psychotherapy and bulimia nervosa: the longer-term effects of interpersonal psychotherapy, behaviour therapy and cognitive behaviour therapy. *Arch Gen Psychiatry.* 1993;50:419–428.

18. Bateman AW, Fonagy P. *Psychotherapy for Borderline Personality Disorder: Mentalization-Based Treatment.* Oxford: Oxford University Press; 2004.

19. Strupp HH, Binder JL. *Psychotherapy in a New Key: A Guide to Time-Limited Dynamic Psychotherapy.* New York: Basic Books; 1984.

20. Gingerich WJ, Eisengart S. Solution-focused brief therapy: a review of the outcome research. *Family Process.* 2000;39:477–498.

21. Miller WR, Rollnick S. *Motivational Interviewing: Preparing People for Change* (2nd ed). New York: Guilford Press; 2002.

Chapter 22

Approaches to stress management

Jon Seskevich

The field of stress management is diverse and encompasses a multitude of different strategies.[1] This chapter will focus on a few valuable approaches that can be used by physicians and other health care providers who care for people facing changes associated with illness.

What is stress?

Stress, in lay terms, is often defined as problems, worries, tension, and pressure. In the context of health, stress can be viewed as dealing with change. Even good changes in life can cause stress. The Social Readjustment Rating Scale, developed by Holmes et al.[2] (Table 22.1), is a convenient and useful tool to estimate the level of stress. Many events that on first appearance do not suggest stress can be stressful. Stress triggers the fight-or-flight response and can cause or contribute to physical problems. Stress hormones can clearly aggravate physical symptoms. Table 22.2 displays the common symptoms triggered by or related to high stress (Table 22.2).[3] Stress management approaches can therefore be used as a form of secondary prevention to reduce the negative impact stress brings to the body.

Table 22.1 The Social Readjustment Rating Scale

Each event should be considered if it has taken place in the last 12 months. Add values to the right of each item to obtain the total score.

Life event	Life change units
Marriage	50
Troubles with the boss	23
Detention in jail or other institution	63
Death of spouse	100
Major change in sleeping habits (a lot more or a lot less sleep, or change in part of day when asleep)	16
Death of a close family member	63
Major change in eating habits (a lot more or a lot less food intake, or very different meal hours or surroundings)	15

Table 22.1 continued	
Foreclosure on a mortgage or loan	30
Revision of personal habits (dress, manners, associations, etc.)	24
Death of a close friend	37
Minor violations of the law (e.g., traffic tickets, jaywalking, disturbing the peace, etc.)	11
Outstanding personal achievement	28
Pregnancy	40
Major change in the health or behavior of a family member	44
Sexual difficulties	39
In-law troubles	29
Major change in number of family get-togethers (e.g., a lot more or a lot less than usual)	15
Major change in financial state (e.g., a lot worse off or a lot better off than usual)	38
Gaining a new family member (e.g., through birth, adoption, elder relative moving in, etc.)	39
Change in residence	20
Son or daughter leaving home (e.g., marriage, attending college, etc.)	29
Marital separation from mate	65
Major change in church activities (e.g., a lot more or a lot less than usual)	19
Marital reconciliation with mate	45
Being fired from work	47
Divorce	73
Changing to a different line of work	36
Major change in the number of arguments with spouse (e.g., a lot more or a lot less than usual regarding childrearing, personal habits, etc.)	35
Major change in responsibilities at work (e.g., promotion, demotion, lateral transfer)	29
Spouse beginning or ceasing work outside the home	26
Major change in working hours or conditions	20
Major change in usual type and/or amount of recreation	19
Taking on a mortgage greater than $10,000 (e.g., purchasing a home, business, etc.)	31
Taking on a mortgage or loan less than $10,000 (e.g., purchasing a car, TV, freezer, etc.)	17
Major personal injury or illness	53
Major business readjustment (e.g., merger, reorganization, bankruptcy, etc.)	39
Major change in social activities (e.g., clubs, dancing, movies, visiting, etc.)	18
Major change in living conditions (e.g., building a new home, remodeling, deterioration of home or neighborhood)	25
Retirement from work	45

Table 22.1 *continued*	
Vacation	13
Christmas	12
Changing to a new school	20
Beginning or ceasing formal schooling	26
Scoring this scale:	
Low	< 149
Mild	150 to 200
Moderate	200 to 299
Major	>300

Due to individual make-up, genetics, utilization of stress coping strategies, health care access, financial reserves, smoking, etc., it is hard to predict who will get an illness due to stress. Higher scores reflect increased risk.

Reprinted from Holmes TH, Rahe RH. The Social Readjustment Rating Scale. *J Psychosom Res.* 1967;11(2):213–218, with permission from Elsevier.

Table 22.2 Self-observable signs of stress

1. General irritability, hyperexcitation, or depression
2. Pounding of the heart
3. Dryness of the throat and mouth
4. Impulsive behavior, emotional instability
5. Overpowering urge to cry or run and hide
6. Inability to concentrate
7. Feeling of unreality, weakness or dizziness
8. Predilection to become fatigued and loss of *joie de vivre*
9. "Floating anxiety"—afraid but not knowing what causes the fear
10. Emotional tension and alertness, feelings of being "keyed up"
11. Trembling, nervous tics
12. Tendency to be easily startled by small sounds, etc.
13. High-pitched, nervous laughter
14. Stuttering and other speech difficulties, which are frequently stress induced
15. Bruxism, or grinding of the teeth
16. Insomnia, usually a consequence of being "keyed up"
17. Hypermotility (technically known as hyperkinesias), the inability to relax
18. Sweating
19. Frequent need to urinate
20. Disturbed gastrointestinal function—diarrhea, indigestion, queasiness and sometimes even vomiting, irritable bowel
21. Migraine headaches
22. Premenstrual tension or missed menstrual cycles
23. Pain in the neck or lower back
24. Loss of or excessive appetite
25. Increased smoking
26. Increased use of legally prescribed drugs, such as tranquilizers or amphetamines
27. Alcohol and drug addiction
28. Nightmares
29. Neurotic behavior
30. Psychoses
31. Accident-proneness

Reprinted with permission from Selye H. *The Stress of Life* (2nd ed.). New York: McGraw-Hill Companies; 1978.

Stress management approaches

It is helpful to keep the patient's personality in mind when approaching the topic of stress management: a one-size-fits-all approach will not work. It is typical to offer advice like, "Relax! Don't worry," but taking such advice is not always easy for humans to do. In the medical context, patients experience a high degree of stress, especially when diagnostic or treatment options are unclear or unknown. A 40-year-old woman said, "Even if it is hospice and I'm going home to die, at least I would know. The waiting is driving me nuts!" One way physicians can alleviate stress is to provide honest information to patients and families as quickly as possible. As the American Cancer Society says, "Knowledge is power." Additionally, encouraging positive coping strategies can potentially mitigate some of the wear and tear that stress can cause.

Receiving support

Even the most independent person will at times need support from others during periods of illness, though accepting help is frequently difficult. A woman hospitalized with metastatic breast cancer and sudden paralysis asked the rounding team if she could see Dr. Kevorkian,[4] as she did not wish to burden others with her illness. She was referred for psychiatric evaluation and stress management and opened up about her work as a volunteer building churches in Central America. When asked how it made her feel to help others, she smiled and said it made her feel good. Asked then how she thought her family might feel if she let them help her, she was able to see that she might not be the burden she had perceived herself to be. She was able to go home shortly after, and her family surrounded her with love and support.

Listening and validating feelings

A skillful physician provides patients with the opportunity to "talk things out." It is important to validate patients' feelings and emotions, maintaining as open and compassionate an attitude as possible. The goal is not to accept or diffuse blame for a circumstance but to acknowledge how difficult the situation (and treatment options) are. Other possible outlets include family members or friends who are willing to listen; professionals such as licensed counselors, social workers, psychologists, psychiatrists, clergy, or nurses; journaling or writing in a diary; or taking advantage of online support resources. Support groups can be excellent strategies. In addition, 12-step groups can help with a variety of challenging problems, including alcohol or drug addiction, overeating, sex addiction, gambling problems, and so forth.

Hope and meaning

Maintaining hope is vital. Viktor Frankl[5] has told of how people with hope were more likely to survive in concentration camps than those who had lost hope. Sometimes, though, the focus of hope needs to shift, especially when goals of treatment are adjusted. For example, a 25-year-old man dying of cancer was seen for stress management. He was obviously grieving. Rather than encourage hope for the unlikely prospect of cure, the discussion focused on the subject of hopes that he still had: pain control, talking with his family, spending quality time with his loved ones. He articulated a hope not to burden his family and to be at home and, if possible, to stay out of the hospital. Encouraging this patient to express his hopes given a known terminal diagnosis facilitated the implementation of strategies to get him home with hospice care.

Stress management techniques

Relaxation techniques
There are many types of relaxation techniques, including conscious breathing, imagery or visualization, progressive muscle relaxation, biofeedback, meditation, and prayer. Different strategies work for different individuals. A woman hospitalized with lupus successfully used visualization, closing her eyes and picturing herself at the beach, seeing the waves come in, feeling the warmth of the sun, and smelling the salt air. She requested that her husband be taught imagery, but despite his efforts he found no benefit from it. He was willing to try another technique and found that progressive muscle relaxation was very effective for him.

A simple but powerful technique involves three steps:

1. Soft belly breathing. Ask the patient to place a hand on the abdomen and breathe softly toward the hand, noticing that the belly gently rises with inhalation and falls with exhalation.
2. Heavy through the body. Ask the patient to let the bed or chair support his or her weight, allowing a feeling of softness, warmth, and heaviness to move through the body.
3. Short, positive word or phrase. Ask the patient to take a meaningful word or phrase and repeat it silently. Remind the patient to kindly and gently let go of any other thoughts and return to the relaxation word or phrase.

With practice, this technique can be used to decrease worry.[6,7]

Activity–rest cycling
In managing chronic pain and other challenging symptoms, an activity–rest plan can prevent exacerbations due to overactivity. With the goal of supporting patients in trying to maximize their productivity, emphasize the importance of an activity–rest plan in an effort to avoid the vicious cycle of pain and inactivity that can result from overdoing it. Suggest alternating periods of activity with rest before the fatigue or pain flares up.[8]

Physical exercise
There is evidence that exercise can be an effective antidepressant.[9] Encourage patients to find something they like to do and to do it regularly. In addition to improving mood, exercise can also ameliorate some underlying health problems.

Spiritual-religious practices
There is a great deal of literature supporting the individual's use of his or her own faith as a positive tool for coping and even improving health outcomes.[10] Do not force your own religious views on a vulnerable patient.

A simple spiritual assessment such as, "Is religion or spirituality important to you? For some it is, for some it isn't. How about you?"[11] can be helpful in determining whether a spiritual approach is appropriate. If yes, a minister or representative from the patient's place of worship can be comforting. Practices such as attending services, prayer, or spiritual study may help spiritually minded patients cope with pain or illness. Hospital chaplains can help patients and families find meaning in their current life experience. Whether the answer is "yes" or "no" to the assessment, all the previous approaches in this chapter can apply.

Good self-care

Just as it is beneficial to work with patients and find stress management practices they can apply to their own lives for improved quality of life and physical functioning, physicians and health care providers will benefit from devoting time and energy to their own well-being. As providers take care of themselves, the quality of their service to others can improve.

References

1. Seaward BL. *Managing Stress: Principles and Strategies for Health and Well-Being* (4th ed). Boston: Jones & Bartlett Publishers; 2004.

2. Holmes TH, Rahe RH. The social readjustment rating scale. *J Psychosom Res.* 1967;2:213–218.

3. Selye H. *The Stress of Life* (2nd ed). New York: McGraw-Hill; 1978:173.

4. Roscoe LA, Malphurs JE, Dragovic LJ, Cohen D. Dr. Jack Kevorkian and cases of euthanasia in Oakland County, Michigan, 1990–1998. *N Engl J Med.* 2000;343:1735–1736.

5. Frankl VE. *Man's Search for Meaning.* Boston: Beacon Press; 1985.

6. Seskevich JE, Crater SW, Lane JD, Krucoff MW. Noetic therapies as adjuncts in stressful medical procedures: beneficial effects on mood prior to percutaneous intervention for unstable coronary syndromes. *Nursing Res.* 2004;53:116–121.

7. Lane JD, Seskevich JE, Pieper CF. Brief meditation training can improve perceived stress and negative mood. *Altern Ther Health Med.* 2007;13:38–44.

8. Gil KM, Ross SL, Keefe FJ. Behavioral treatment of chronic pain: four pain management protocols. In: France RD, Krishnan KR, eds. *Chronic pain.* New York: American Psychiatric Press; 1988:376–413.

9. Blumenthal JA, Babyak MA, Doraiswamy PM, Watkins L. Exercise and pharmacotherapy in the treatment of major depressive disorder. *Psychosom Med.* 2007;69:587–596.

10. Koenig HG. Religion, spirituality, and medicine: research findings and implications for clinical practice. *South Med J.* 2004;97:1194–1200.

11. Seskevich JE. Assessing spirituality with grace. *Integrative Nursing.* 2003;2:12.

Chapter 23

Neurocognitive and psychological assessment

Guy G. Potter

Clinical scenario

M.D. is an 82-year-old retired physician brought to the ED by his wife and son, who request nursing home placement for him. He is admitted to the psychiatry service. This is his second admission in 6 months. M.D. has a long history of chronic depression and substance abuse, including prescription medication abuse. His depression has been treated with a number of antidepressants, as well as lithium, benzodiazepines, and trials of atypical antipsychotics. Lately his family has been concerned about his decreasing cognitive function. Even though he has been enrolled in a day program, his wife and son feel his cognitive decline is so pronounced that they can no longer care for him at home.

M.D. is adamantly opposed to nursing home placement and begs constantly to be released home. He reports fatigue, anhedonia, and apathy. He states that he enjoys singing and listening to music, but the church choir practices only once a week. He cannot provide an answer as to why he is unable to listen to music at home. He repeatedly demands medications to help him sleep, as well as medications to give him more energy.

Mental status examination reveals a slim, kempt older man with normal affect. Psychomotor behavior is notable for some increased activity, moving from sitting to lying position repeatedly throughout the interview. Thought process is circumstantial, with obsession and perseveration regarding his symptoms and request for medications. His Mini-Mental State Examination (MMSE) is scored at 26/30. His insight and judgment are limited.

The following factors present unique challenges in the accurate assessment of M.D.:

1. With this MMSE score, is M.D. capable of making an appropriate decision for his health needs such that legal guardianship and placement in a skilled facility is appropriate?
2. Are M.D.'s cognitive symptoms attributable to depression or other psychiatric illness, or are they related to either a primary cognitive disorder or the initial manifestations of dementia?

3. Are there drug-seeking behaviors or maladaptive personality characters playing significant roles in his clinical manifestations?

Referral for neuropsychological evaluation can be appropriate in situations such as this one where there is a clinical or diagnostic dilemma, and where issues of cognitive change, psychiatric disturbance, decision-making capacity, or secondary gain may be playing a role.

Background

A neuropsychological evaluation assesses both neurocognitive and psychological functions by using test instruments designed to yield results that are both reliable and valid. Neurocognitive functions such as memory, attention, and problem solving have underlying neural substrates that can be compromised by numerous medical or psychiatric conditions,[1] and medical illnesses are often associated with neural changes leading to depression, anxiety, and other alterations in mood or behavior.[2] Psychological functions including acute emotional state, personality variables, and motivation may contribute to neurocognitive performance; however, there are also a number of cases in which specific psychological symptoms are indicative of a medical or neurological disorder and merit a stand-alone assessment. Medical conditions that are comorbid with neurocognitive or psychological dysfunction can be a source of excess disability and can complicate treatment outcomes. Neurocognitive and psychological dysfunction should be assessed carefully because many patients lack accurate perception or even awareness of their deficits, and a reliable and valid characterization of a patient's function in these areas is an important aid to diagnosis and treatment planning.

Neurocognitive assessment

Most clinical tests of neurocognitive function have been developed in the field of neuropsychology, which specializes in diagnosing and treating the neurocognitive and behavioral manifestations of brain dysfunction. The validity of neurocognitive test instruments is based on their ability to assess the neurocognitive functions they purport to assess. For example, a memory test is expected to (1) detect memory dysfunction and produce results consistent with other tests or neuroimaging markers of abnormal memory, and (2) detect impairment among individuals with known memory disorders. A reliable neuropsychological test is expected to produce similar results when scored or administered by different individuals, to provide consistent results when stable neurocognitive functions are assessed at different time points, and to detect positive and negative changes in performance consistent with changes in underlying neurobiological processes. Reliability and validity are achieved in part by the use of standardized administration and scoring procedures. Neuropsychological test results are adjusted for age, sex, education, and ethnicity, which are potential modifiers of test outcome. Attention to these principles of test development allows neurocognitive measures to assess a wide range of neurocognitive abilities with greater sensitivity and specificity than bedside tests such as the Folstein Mini-Mental State Examination (MMSE),[3] which are used for global neurocognitive screening but lack sufficient item content to thoroughly assess individual neurocognitive domains. The objectivity and scientific grounding of neuropsychological testing provides confidence that results obtained from a neuropsychological evaluation are less influenced by demographic variables or subjective impressions, and instead provide a reflection of the patient's underlying cognition and brain function.

Psychological assessment and symptom validity

Psychological testing is typically included in a neuropsychological evaluation and helps a clinician estimate the extent to which acute emotional state, personality variables, and motivation may contribute to neurocognitive performance. For instance, psychological testing may highlight personality disorders or character tendencies that present challenges to treatment. Psychological assessment can also aid in the differential diagnosis of psychiatric disorders by providing additional data about the presence of features such as psychoticism, mania, somatization, or malingering. In some contexts, illness or disability may have financial or emotional advantages for an individual, and it is important to evaluate the possibility of feigned neurocognitive or psychiatric symptoms, whether they are intentional (e.g., malingering) or unintentional (e.g., somatoform spectrum). Neuropsychological and psychological assessment may include tests or indices of symptom validity, which are typically based on identifying patterns of test performance, behavior, or symptom endorsement that are highly anomalous or improbable relative to known principles of neurocognitive, neurological, or psychiatric function. Many personality inventories, for instance, have scales that are sensitive to over- and under-reporting of symptoms. Although concern about symptom validity may render neuropsychological or psychological testing invalid if it presents a sufficient confound to test interpretation, it may also identify individuals who are not candid about their neurocognitive or psychiatric symptoms.

Objective psychological tests are typically multidimensional self-report questionnaires that assess a range of emotional, cognitive, and personality characteristics. They are used much more frequently in a medical setting than are projective tests; however, both types of testing require trained clinical interpretation and should be used in conjunction with a clinical interview.

The process of neurocognitive-psychological testing

A neuropsychological evaluation includes diagnostic interviewing, behavioral observations, and assessment of neurocognitive performance. The objectives and content of the interview are similar to other psychiatric and medical interviews, but with attention to issues that may influence neurocognitive and psychological function. Important features to elicit in a neuropsychological evaluation include the following:

- Medical history, with particular attention to head injuries, substance use, and potential neurotoxic exposures
- Educational history, probing for evidence of longstanding learning disorders that may confound diagnosis of acquired impairments
- Occupational history, which surveys job duties to (1) estimate premorbid function and (2) estimate how neurocognitive impairment may affect future work performance
- Behavioral observations, which provide the clinician with an opportunity to assess behaviors suggestive of particular brain disorders. For instance, many behavioral aspects of frontal lobe dysfunction (e.g., disinhibition, perseveration, stimulus bound behaviors) can be elicited in an interview. Behavioral observations also include identifying difficulties in vision, hearing, or motor function that may complicate testing or exacerbate neurocognitive difficulties.

Neuropsychological assessment in a medical setting requires consideration of how physical difficulties such as fatigue or pain may affect the patient's performance. Neuropsychological evaluation of acutely ill patients may take less than 60 minutes and sample neurocognitive abilities to the extent that broad questions about areas of impairment can be addressed; in healthier patients, 3 to 6 hours of evaluation may be needed to obtain a comprehensive assessment of neurocognitive strengths and weaknesses sufficient to answer multiple, complex referral questions.

Table 23.1 Areas assessed in neuropsychological evaluation accompanied by representative neurocognitive measures

Neuropsychological domains	Representative neurocognitive measures
Premorbid ability	Wechsler Test of Adult Reading
Orientation	Benton Temporal Orientation
Intelligence	Wechsler Adult Intelligence Scale (WAIS-III)
Attention span	WAIS-III Digit Span subtest
Sustained attention	Connors' Continuous Performance Test
Complex attention	Trail Making Test
Processing speed	Symbol-Digit Modalities Test
Problem solving	Wisconsin Card Sorting Test
Verbal learning	California Verbal Learning Test-2
Nonverbal learning	Brief Visuospatial Naming Test-Revised
Word retrieval/naming	Boston Naming Test
Verbal fluency	Letter fluency (FAS), category fluency (Animal Naming)
Visual-spatial processing	Judgment of Line Orientation, Rey Complex Figure
Motor speed/coordination	Finger Tapping, Grooved Pegboard
Symptom validity	Word Memory Test, Test of Memory Malingering
Psychological	Minnesota Multiphasic Personality Inventory-2

With respect to individual differences, neuropsychologists attempt to avoid tests that are too hard or too easy for the patient's functional level, as either case can lead to false-negative or false-positive errors in diagnosing impairment. Table 23.1 describes the functions assessed in a neuropsychological evaluation.

Indications for obtaining neurocognitive and/ or psychological assessment

There are three major applications of neurocognitive testing in medical settings:

1. Detecting brain dysfunction via characterization of both normal and abnormal neurocognitive performance
2. Informing clinical care decisions with respect to functional abilities and intervention approaches
3. Tracking changes in cognitive performance over time or as a result of specific treatment interventions

Neuropsychological testing provides information for differential diagnosis based on the performance ranges of a test, as well as on the pattern of performances among tests. In a medical setting, the need for a neuropsychological evaluation may occur when bedside neurocognitive testing such as the MMSE is consistent with impairment (as in dementia) but there is not enough information to estimate the nature of the impairment (such as Alzheimer's disease versus vascular dementia or depression). Neuropsychologists are often called upon to provide supplementary data on whether deficits in abilities such as problem-solving, information processing speed, or visual processing might compromise functional activities such as money management,[4] driving,[5] or decision-making capacity.[6]

Serial neuropsychological assessments may track patients with comorbid medical illness to assess the effect of treatment on neurocognitive function. Neurocognitive deficits associated with a medical condition may mask an underlying cognitive impairment or dementia, and follow-up assessments can help assess the extent to which baseline neurocognitive deficits are reversible (as in some depression and many metabolic and endocrine abnormalities), stable (as in many cerebrovascular events), or progressive (as in Alzheimer's disease and other dementias) in nature.

The case of M.D. highlights some reasons to obtain neurocognitive and psychological assessment: (1) there is a question about differential diagnosis of cognitive function, (2) there are questions about discharge placement that may be influenced by neurocognitive and psychological disorder, and (3) his status may need to be reassessed in the future after treatment of acute psychiatric and medical issues. As illustrated here, a consultation for neuropsychological assessment is most efficient when there are specific referral questions to guide the neuropsychologist in selecting the most effective battery of tests.

Using the neuropsychological report in clinical decision-making

The neuropsychological report, the product of the neuropsychological evaluation, includes the following:

1. Description of data collected (relevant medical, psychiatric, and psychosocial history; behavioral observations; test results)
2. Interpretation of the data in terms of neurocognitive functioning and diagnostic impressions
3. Relevant recommendations for cognitive rehabilitation, compensation strategies, psychotherapy, and other treatment issues

Test results are informative for treatment providers who seek in-depth data and statistical performance measures, while the interpretation section (e.g., Summary and Impressions) integrates the test results with all other clinical data obtained. Although neurocognitive test scores are the primary source of data in a neuropsychological evaluation, interpretation involves integrating test performances with information from the diagnostic interview and behavioral observations, as well as the neuropsychologist's training in neuroanatomy, cognition, behavior disorders, and neurobehavioral diagnosis. This includes accounting for factors such as motivation, depression, or anxiety that may pose caveats to interpretation. Neuropsychological interpretation may also entail excluding diagnoses that are not consistent with a patient's presentation and testing.

Recommendations for clinical care are based on the pattern of strengths and weaknesses in test performances; for instance, characteristics of observed memory deficits may lead to specific memory strategies to help an individual remember medications or appointments.

Return to clinical scenario

The neuropsychological assessment for M.D. showed that his pattern of performance was consistent with a descriptive diagnosis of "cognitive impairment, not demented." Results indicated a pattern of slowed information processing speed and executive dysfunction, but with preserved temporal orientation and memory storage as evidenced by errorless recognition memory. Test results suggested that depression was likely a prominent contributor to his neurocognitive deficits, although other causes such as multiple medications, hypertension, and history of alcohol and narcotics might be exacerbating his current cognitive difficulties.

The treating physicians and M.D. decided to pursue electroconvulsive therapy (ECT) for treatment of depression. M.D.'s presenting symptoms improved after four ECT sessions, and he showed significant reduction of drug seeking, increased energy, and increased initiative in his daily activities; however, he also continued to demonstrate mild neurocognitive difficulties. He was discharged to his family and continued to attend his day program. M.D.'s medical and psychiatric histories suggest elevated risk for persistent cognitive impairment or dementia, and longitudinal neuropsychological assessment is recommended every 1 to 2 years to track the extent to which the observed neurocognitive deficits are reversible, stable, or progressive in nature.

Summary

A neuropsychological evaluation provides a standardized and objective assessment of neurocognitive and psychological functions that is sensitive to individual differences in age, sex, ethnicity, and education. It can provide important information for diagnosis and treatment planning in a medical setting.

References

1. Houston WS, Bondi MW. Potentially reversible cognitive symptoms in older adults. In: Attix DK, Welsh-Bohmer KA, eds. *Geriatric Neuropsychology: Assessment and Intervention.* New York: Guilford; 2006:103–129.

2. Pomeroy C, Mitchell JE, Roerig J, Crow S. *Medical Complications of Psychiatric Illnesses.* Washington, DC: American Psychiatric Publishing; 2002.

3. Folstein M, Folstein S, Fanjiang G. *Mini-Mental State Examination: Clinical Guide and User's Guide.* Lutz, FL: Psychological Assessment Resources; 2001.

4. Cahn-Weiner DA, Farias ST, Julian L, et al. Cognitive and neuroimaging predictors of instrumental activities of daily living. *J Int Neuropsychol Soc.* 2007;13(5):747–757.

5. Lesikar SE, Gallo JJ, Rebok GW, Keyl PM. Prospective study of brief neuropsychological measures to assess crash risk in older primary care patients. *J Am Board Fam Pract.* 2002;15(1):11–19.

6. Marson D, Hebert KR. Functional assessment. In: Attix DK, Welsh-Bohmer KA, eds. *Geriatric Neuropsychology: Assessment and Intervention.* New York: Guilford; 2006:158–197.

Index

169